healthy eating
for prostate care

Professor Margaret Rayman,
Kay Dilley, and Kay Gibbons

PROSTATE CANCER RESEARCH FOUNDATION

healthy eating for prostate care

Photography by Will Heap

Kyle Books

This edition published in 2009 by Kyle
Books, an imprint of Kyle Cathie Limited
www.kylecathie.com

Distributed by National Book Network
4501 Forbes Blvd., Suite 200, Lanham,
MD20706

ISBN 978-1-906868-04-8

Editor Katharina Hahn
Editorial assistant Vicki Murrell
Designer Arno Devo
Photographer Will Heap
Proofreader Anne Newman
Indexer Alex Corrin
Americanizer Delora Jones
Home economist and stylist
  Annie Nichols
Production Lisa Pinnell, Gemma John

A catalog record for this book is available
from the Library of Congress.

Color reproduction by Sang Choy
Printed in Singapore by Star Standard

contents

acknowledgments

Our grateful thanks go to celebrity chefs Raymond Blanc, Gino D'Acampo, Alex Mackay, Cyrus Todiwala, and Antony Worrall Thompson for providing us with some wonderful recipes. Particular thanks go to John Walter, Head Chef at the University of Surrey's Lakeside Restaurant, who searched his repertoire for dishes to fulfill our rigorous criteria, and to Dr. John Rayman who tried and tested many recipes and contributed a number of his own.

We are also most grateful for the expert help provided by Professor Peter Bramley (lycopene), Professor Mike Clifford (polyphenols), Dr. Jonathan Brown (phytoestrogens), Dr. Albena Dinkova-Kostova (cruciferous vegetables), and Dr. John Lodge (vitamin E), who checked the scientific text for accuracy, and to Dr. Elina Hyppönen and Professor Joe Millward, who gave helpful advice on vitamin D.

Last but not least, we would like to thank our friends and families who both provided recipes and supported and encouraged us throughout this very demanding project.

Disclaimer: The information in this book is the authors' best interpretation of the scientific literature at the time of going to press. Following the guidelines given is no guarantee of benefit in reducing the risk or preventing the spread of prostate cancer.

foreword by the PCRF

The Prostate Cancer Research Foundation (PCRF) has two aims: first, to promote independent worldwide research into all aspects of prostate cancer, and second, to share the crucial knowledge gathered from that research via our Forum, which is attended by the world's top prostate cancer experts.

Our objectives are:
* To fund research that helps to find the cure for prostate cancer.
* To fund research that contributes to finding the causes of prostate cancer.
* To fund the best quality research.
* To fund research that offers better outcomes to men who are diagnosed with prostate cancer.
* To enable prostate cancer specialists to share information on a regular basis.

Why research is so important
Prostate cancer is the most common form of cancer in men in the United States, with over 185,000 new cases reported in 2008. It is the second-most common cause of cancer-deaths in men in the United States, with over 28,000 deaths in 2008, according to the National Cancer Institute.

More research into the disease is needed, as there is still so much we do not know. For example, we do not know why the prostate enlarges in a benign manner as men grow older. We do not have an accurate test that differentiates between cancers that need urgent treatment and those cancers that may never need treating. Funding for research into prostate cancer is significantly less than for other common cancers, but the need is greater than ever as the incidence is estimated to increase sharply as our population ages.

The PCRF has been proud to support Professor Rayman since 2004, when we first funded her project to investigate the effects of selenium intake and its ability to reduce the incidence of prostate cancer. This initial research has led to the development of this cookbook.

Evidence clearly points to diet as a significant factor in the development of prostate cancer, and several studies have reported increased prostate cancer in populations that have switched from their traditional diet to a Western one. However, despite these instances, there has never been a study to combine all the published research on diet and the implications for prostate cancer development. This cookbook is a unique and valuable resource for men and their families who would like to put these findings to practical use and help in maintaining a healthy prostate. The recipes included in this book by Professor Rayman and her team can help men understand the types of foods that may be beneficial, and in what quantities.

We are very pleased to be able to support this cookbook and we know it will become a very valuable resource for men, and for those who care about them, to help improve the health of their prostates.

Bon Appetit!

Dr. Chris Adams, Chairman
Professor Christopher Woodhouse, Scientific Chairman

introduction

Rarely a day passes without new claims being made of the beneficial or harmful effects of diet on health and disease. The claims made for prostate cancer are no exception. There is growing scientific evidence that strongly suggests that diets rich in certain foods can help prevent this disease or its spread. There is also evidence to indicate a harmful effect of other foods. Prostate cancer is often slow to develop and spread and so, strategies that can influence its progression have considerable potential. For those living with the condition, a controlled diet may provide the only means of active treatment. But it can be hard to interpret the evidence and put it into practice. Here we have untangled the scientific jargon and put all the information into one place to enable you to benefit from this research. By simply following our recommendations and including some of these tried and tested recipes in your diet, you could improve the health of your prostate.

The scale of the prostate cancer problem
A hundred and eighty thousand new diagnoses each year in the US make prostate cancer the most common cancer to affect American men. About 1 in 6 American men will be diagnosed with prostate cancer at some point, but only about 1 in 35 men will die of it, according to the American Cancer Society. Prostate cancer has become more common over the last two decades, though this is partly due to more widespread screening and improved detection techniques. On a global scale, prostate cancer is the second-most common cancer after lung cancer. The numbers vary greatly between countries, with the highest rates reported in the US and Sweden, and the lowest in Japan, India, and China. This reported variation may also be partly due to differences in the availability of screening and detection techniques, but it is widely accepted that at least some of it is due to differences in diet.

What are the risk factors?
The causes of prostate cancer are not fully understood, but there are several known risk factors, the greatest of which is age, with risk increasing rapidly from 50 onwards. The existence of prostate cancer or breast cancer in an immediate family member also increases risk. Men of African-American descent appear to have an increased risk while men of Asian descent have a lower risk. These risk factors cannot be modified. There is, however, a growing body of evidence to show that there is a major risk factor which can be modified —that of diet.

Diet—a modifiable risk factor
The link between diet and prostate cancer is reflected in the low disease rates in Asian countries where diets are low in meat and saturated fats, and high in plant foods, fiber, and fish. This contrasts with the high rates in Western countries where diets are rich in meat and fat, and low in plant foods. When people migrate from an Asian country to a Western country and adopt the diet and lifestyle of that country, their risk of prostate cancer increases. Furthermore, the incidence of cancer in Asia is increasing with Westernization. This strengthens the theory that development of prostate cancer is affected by environmental factors, the most important of which is probably diet. There are several nutrients and foods which research shows may be able to influence the risk of prostate cancer development and progression, making dietary modification a useful and accessible strategy. It is important to remember, however, that research in all these areas is ongoing, and the picture may very well change as more information becomes available.

How can foods and nutrients affect the risk of prostate cancer development and progression?
Research has shown that some nutrients and food components can act through one or a combination of the mechanisms summarized below to reduce the risk and spread of cancer. A full explanation of these mechanisms can be found in the Second Expert Report of the World Cancer Research Fund American Institute for Cancer Research "Food, Nutrition, Physical Activity, and the Prevention of Cancer: a Global Perspective," which can be accessed on www.dietandcancerreport. org.

Some foods or nutrients may:
* behave as antioxidants, reducing oxidative stress that can damage cells and molecules
* reduce inflammation which is associated with a higher risk of cancer
* improve the immune response, helping the body fight cancer

* prevent damage to DNA or help its repair
* halt the growth of prostate cancer cells
* cause prostate cancer cells to die
* reduce the invasion of tumor cells into the surrounding tissue
* prevent the formation of new blood vessels in the tumor, reducing its ability to grow
* change the behavior of genes so that protective genes can act efficiently
* increase the rate at which compounds that can cause cancer can be detoxified and removed from the body
* modify the behavior of hormones or their receptors, most notably by reducing the activation of the androgen receptor which can reduce prostate cancer risk.

(See Glossary on page 170 for explanation of terms used)

Identifying the relevant foods and the quantities required

Through extensive reading of the published literature on the topic, we have identified foods and nutrients that have been linked to prostate cancer, both beneficially and detrimentally. These foods and food components are listed in the table below. The evidence for each of these foods and nutrients is discussed separately in the following pages. Research is ongoing but the most convincing evidence is probably that for lycopene/tomatoes and selenium.

Evidence for an effect of these foods is provided by studies carried out on human populations. In these studies, intakes of the food in question or levels in the blood are recorded within a population group and compared to rates of prostate cancer. In this way, it is possible to identify whether high intakes of a certain food are associated with an increased or decreased risk.

Further evidence can be seen in animal studies, but it is hard to draw direct comparisons with humans. Finally, interesting observations have been made in laboratory experiments where food components or nutrients have been added to prostate cancer cells. These studies provide an insight into the effects of each food component.

For each food or food component identified, we endeavored to establish the quantity required in the diet for a noticeable effect. Based on this, and taking into account a realistic level of intake, we have made recommendations for consumption or limitation in the diet. Quantitative guidelines have been given where possible.

To help increase intake and meet these guidelines, we have selected recipes that are rich in the foods and nutrients believed to be beneficial for protecting against prostate cancer. For each recipe, we have indicated which beneficial foods or nutrients are well represented in that dish; see "good source of" for substantial amounts and "source of" for smaller but significant amounts. In setting these measures, we have considered the number of times per day that a food is likely to be eaten, as well as the amount that is realistic to use in a recipe. For further information, the approximate calorie, fat, and saturated fat content of each portion has also been included.

Taking control

In addition to the potential physical benefits of changing your diet, using this cookbook may have psychological benefits. Consciously making changes

Foods and nutrients linked with a beneficial or detrimental effect on prostate cancer risk	
Beneficial	**Detrimental**
Allium vegetables	Burnt or overcooked meat
Cruciferous vegetables	Dairy products
Fish	Fat and saturated fat
Tomatoes/Lycopene	
Phytoestrogens	
Polyphenols	
Selenium	
Vitamin D	
Vitamin E	

to your diet and lifestyle is associated with a positive, optimistic attitude and a feeling of being in control. This has long been known to improve the immune system and can therefore have a direct effect on how your disease progresses. Men with an increasing PSA level after primary treatment, who attended a series of dietary and cooking classes, were able to make a change to a prostate-healthy diet that emphasized plant-based foods and fish. Three months later, their PSA doubling time had lengthened and quality of life had improved. We hope that this book will empower many men and their families to be active participants in influencing the outcome of their disease.

One last word

While the evidence for an effect of many of these foods on prostate cancer risk or spread, when taken separately, may be inconclusive, when taken together their effect may be significant. Food components can interact so that the effect they have together is more than the sum of their individual effects; for instance, components of soy can intensify the ability of vitamin D to slow the growth of prostate cancer cells. With that in mind, even if you cannot achieve the full recommendations, we encourage you to attempt as many of the suggested modifications to your diet as possible.

allium vegetables

Allium vegetables are bulbous plants that have a distinctive taste and odor that make them ideal for use in cooking. Commonly eaten *Allium* vegetables include garlic, onion, scallions (spring onions), shallots, leeks, and chives. Some research suggests that men who eat a diet rich in these foods have a lower risk of developing prostate cancer.

The taste and odor of *Allium* vegetables comes from a group of organosulphur compounds. These are formed during the natural aging process of the plant or from the activity of an enzyme called alliinase that is released when the plant is chopped or crushed. It is these compounds that have been identified as having anti-cancer properties. It is important to note, however, as shown with garlic, that the heat of cooking can destroy alliinase activity, preventing the formation of the active anti-cancer compounds. However, if garlic is left sitting for 10 minutes after cutting or crushing, the alliinase has time to do its work and the active allyl sulphur compounds are formed.

Evidence from human studies

Garlic is the *Allium* vegetable most commonly described in research studies as having anti-cancer properties. A small Turkish study demonstrated a reduction in PSA level in nine patients with prostate cancer after they had taken a liquid garlic extract for a period of one month. The average PSA level of these men fell from 8.9 to 3.6ng/ml, and the fall was accompanied by an improvement in symptoms.

A study carried out in Shanghai investigated the effect of intake of *Allium* vegetables, including garlic, scallions, onions, chives, and leeks, on the risk of prostate cancer in 238 men with confirmed prostate cancer, and 471 healthy men for comparison. Results showed that men who ate more than 10g (1/3 ounce) of *Allium* vegetables per day were 49 percent less likely to develop prostate cancer than those who ate less than 2.2g per day. When vegetables were considered individually, men who ate more than 2.1g of garlic or scallions (spring onions) per day reduced their risk of developing the disease by 53 percent (garlic) and 70 percent (scallions) compared to those who did not eat garlic or scallions at all.

While some studies have seen a protective association between *Allium* vegetables and the risk of prostate cancer, others have seen none. This may be partly due to the varied types and concentrations of organosulphur compounds but may also reflect the fact that formation of the active compounds takes time to occur and is prevented if the vegetables are cooked immediately after preparation. *Allium* vegetables are also often served with other foods, such as tomatoes, that have been identified as having anti-cancer properties so the effect may be from the combination rather than from one type of vegetable alone.

The effect of *Allium* vegetables

Allium vegetables or their products, e.g., diallyl disulphide (DADS), are reported to suppress the activation of cancer-causing compounds, increase the action of enzymes that detoxify cancer-causing compounds, prevent the growth of new blood vessels that are required for the tumor to grow, suppress cancer cell division, cause the death of cancer cells, decrease DNA damage, and reduce the response to androgen. They have also been shown to help reduce inflammation, a feature associated with many cancers.

Other components of garlic and onion, besides organosulphur compounds, are said to have cancer-preventative effects. For instance, garlic is a source of the amino acid arginine, which may help to reduce inflammation, while onions are a source of the polyphenol, quercetin, which can help prevent cancer-cell growth.

What quantity of *Allium* vegetables do we eat?

The quantities of onion and garlic consumed by population groups in ten European countries were reported by the European Prospective Investigation into Cancer and Nutrition (EPIC) in 2002. Men in Greece were reported to eat the largest amount of onions and garlic with an average daily intake of over 28g, while men in Germany were reported to eat the least, with an average daily serving of less than 8g. The average intake of onion and garlic by the general population of the UK is reported as being less than 10g per day, with only 15 percent of British males eating 6g (about 2 cloves) or more of garlic per week, compared to 46 percent of Shanghai men.

The average use of onions in America was reported by the United States Department of Agriculture (USDA) as being 21.6 lb. per person per year in 2006 (equivalent to about an ounce a day). The USDA also reported that the American demand for garlic had increased during the 1990s along with greater awareness of its potential health benefits. Garlic use in 2008 was estimated as 3 lb. per person, equivalent to about 3.7g (about 1/10 ounce) per day which was more than double the use recorded in 1990.

Other benefits and risks of *Allium* vegetables

Other health benefits attributed to garlic and onions include protection against microbial infections and the reduction of risk factors for cardiovascular disease. While *Allium* vegetables are generally safe to consume, it should be noted that garlic is known to have a thinning effect on blood and can interfere with some prescription drugs.

Recommendations

The current UK guideline for fruit and vegetable consumption is at least five 80g (3-ounce) portions per day. In the US, 2–2½ cups of vegetables per day are recommended. Although there are no specific guidelines for the consumption of *Allium* vegetables, the World Health Organization (WHO) suggests 2–5g (approximately one clove) of fresh garlic per day for general health promotion in adults. We suggest that you consume *Allium* vegetables, particularly garlic, several times per week. Don't forget that garlic should be left sitting for about 10 minutes after crushing or chopping it before you cook it to allow the anti-cancer compounds time to form.

The summary table below details the quantities of *Allium* vegetables associated with beneficial effects, as well as our suggested target intake and our definition of a "good source of" and "source of" that have been included in the recipes in the book.

Allium Vegetables	
Effects seen at... (depending on the study)	Greater than 10g (¹/₃ ounce) of *Allium* vegetables per day *or* greater than 2.1g of garlic or scallions per day
Target intake...	3 or more garlic cloves per week *or* 3 or more servings of 3 ounces *Allium* vegetables per week
Good source of...	1 clove of garlic 3 ounces *Allium* vegetables
Source of...	¼ clove of garlic ²/₃ ounce *Allium* vegetables

cruciferous vegetables

Cruciferous vegetables are edible plants from the *Cruciferae (Brassicaceae)* family that take their name from their flower which has four petals in a cross-like shape. The most commonly eaten cruciferous vegetables are listed below:

* Broccoli
* Cauliflower
* Cabbage
* Brussels sprouts
* Bok choy (Pak choi)
* Arugula
* Watercress
* Collard
* Kale
* Radish
* Turnip
* Garden cress
* Mustard
* Rutabaga (Swede)
* Horseradish
* Wasabi

All cruciferous vegetables contain compounds known as glucosinolates. When the vegetables are bruised, chopped, or chewed, the enzyme myrosinase is released from the broken cells and reacts with the glucosinolates to form compounds known as isothiocyanates and indoles. It is these sulphur-containing compounds that are responsible for the sometimes pungent aroma and spicy taste of these vegetables. More importantly, they are biologically active and have been identified as having anti-cancer properties.

Because the activity of myrosinase is destroyed upon heating, cooking can prevent the conversion of glucosinolates to the desirable isothiocyanate and indole products; for instance, microwave cooking or rapid boiling have been shown to completely destroy myrosinase activity. It is also important to note that because glucosinolates are water soluble, they can leach into cooking water and are lost if it is discarded.

Some gut bacteria are known to produce myrosinase, allowing glucosinolates to be converted to isothiocyanates when cruciferous vegetables are digested. Some people's gut bacteria are more efficient at doing this than others, allowing them to derive more benefit from cooked cruciferous vegetables. In situations where gut bacteria are being reduced or eliminated, for instance during prolonged antibiotic intake, the health benefits from cruciferous vegetables will be much reduced. On top of that, some people are more genetically predisposed than others to benefit from eating cruciferous vegetables: these individuals cannot produce one or more of the enzymes that break down isothiocyanates so they eliminate them more slowly and are therefore exposed to their beneficial effects for a longer time.

Evidence from human studies

Cruciferous vegetables contain a number of different glucosinolates at varying concentrations. Those that have been identified as potentially beneficial can be found in broccoli, brussels sprouts, cabbage, cauliflower, kale, watercress, and arugula. Furthermore, it appears that sprouts from broccoli seed contain the beneficial compounds in greater concentration than in the fully grown broccoli plant itself.

A recently published study of fruit and vegetable intake found a strong association between consumption of cruciferous vegetables and reductions in prostate-cancer risk. The study population, a group of more than 29,000 predominantly white males, had a 40 percent decrease in risk of extraprostatic cancer, (defined as stage III or IV), if they were in the group that consumed the most cruciferous vegetables compared to those who consumed the least. The highest-intake group consumed on average 1.1 servings of cruciferous vegetables per day, while the lowest-intake group only consumed an average of 0.1 servings per day. These servings were defined as one cup of leafy vegetables or one-half cup of other vegetables such as broccoli and cauliflower. Furthermore, when the vegetables were considered individually, those who ate broccoli or cauliflower more than once a week had a 45 percent (broccoli) or 52 percent (cauliflower) lower risk of extraprostatic cancer and a 24 percent (broccoli) reduction in risk for aggressive prostate cancer, defined as stage III or IV, or Gleason score (see Glossary) greater or equal to 7, than those who ate them less than once per month.

Despite the impressive findings of a number of studies, much of the evidence has been inconsistent. This may be partly due to the problems associated with the assessment of dietary intake of cruciferous vegetables, such as the limitation of accuracy associated with recalling past intake of foods. Furthermore, as previously mentioned, the glucosinolate content of cruciferous vegetables can vary in both type and concentration, can be lost during cooking, and can have a more pronounced effect on certain individuals.

How do cruciferous vegetables work?

Isothiocyanates and indoles probably act by a number of mechanisms in the prevention and inhibition of prostate cancer. Some of the actions appear to be unique to specific compounds, while others are common to more than one compound. Effects include reduced growth and increased death of cancer cells, lower activation of androgen receptors, less invasion of cancer cells into surrounding tissues, reduced inflammation, and the detoxification and removal of cancer-causing compounds.

What amount of cruciferous vegetables do we eat?

The International Agency for Research on Cancer reported in 2004 that cruciferous vegetables such as cabbage, broccoli, cauliflower, brussels sprouts, and watercress appeared to account for 10–15 percent of total vegetable intake. Consumption varied across Europe with intakes of around 1 ounce per day in some northern European countries and less than ½ ounce per day in the south. The average intake in North America was reported to be 1 ounce per day, with the highest consumption—more than 3½ ounces per day—in China.

Other benefits and risks of eating cruciferous vegetables

Some studies have shown that cruciferous vegetables can lower the risk of coronary heart disease and stroke, and reduce inflammation, a factor in many diseases.

Certain cruciferous vegetables, notably broccoli, have a high content of vitamin K, which has a role in blood coagulation. Interactions have been seen with warfarin medication but only at intakes much higher than our recommendations. As a note of caution however, cruciferous vegetables can interfere with the uptake of the mineral iodine by the thyroid gland, resulting in growth of the thyroid. Reassuringly, however, a clinical study found no adverse effects. Nonetheless, it would be prudent to ensure an adequate supply of iodine in the diet to avoid straining the thyroid. The richest sources of dietary iodine are seafood and fish but we would also recommend the use of iodized salt in place of regular salt.

Recommendations

There are no specific guidelines for the consumption of cruciferous vegetables apart from the general guidelines for fruit and vegetable consumption. Research suggests that the risk of prostate cancer is reduced with regular consumption of cruciferous vegetables. It may therefore be beneficial to choose one of the cruciferous vegetables, particularly broccoli, brussels sprouts, cabbage, cauliflower, kale, watercress, or arugula, as one of your daily servings of vegetables, or to include them at least several times per week. You may be able to find broccoli sprouts (or sprout the seeds yourself at home) to add to salads, sandwiches, or stir-fries. It is also important to remember that to retain as many of the beneficial compounds as possible, cruciferous vegetables should be eaten raw (e.g., coleslaw), or only lightly cooked using cooking methods that use less water, such as steaming.

The summary table to the right details the quantities of cruciferous vegetables consumed in studies where beneficial effects have been noted, as well as our suggested target intake and our definition of a "good source of" and "source of" as used for recipes in the book.

Cruciferous Vegetables

Effects seen at... (according to human studies)	More than 3 servings of cruciferous vegetables per week up to 1 serving of cruciferous vegetables per day *or* 2 servings per week of broccoli or cauliflower
Target intake...	3–5 3-ounce servings of cruciferous vegetables per week
Good source of...	3 ounces
Source of...	$2/3$ ounce

fish

The oils present in cold-water fish belong to a group of fats known as omega-3 fatty acids. Although omega-3 fatty acids are also found in plants and plant foods (notably in flaxseed/linseed, rapeseed, canola, and walnut), they are the short-chain form, which is not easily usable by the body. By contrast, oily fish contain pre-formed, long-chain, omega-3 fatty acids. These fats are essential for human health with known roles in vision, the immune system, and brain function, and they appear to protect against sudden cardiac death. Rates of prostate cancer are low in parts of the world, such as Asia, where oily fish consumption is high, leading to the suggestion that fish or fish oils may have protective effects against the disease.

Evidence from human studies

Though studies in animals and experiments in laboratories show that fish oils have the potential to reduce the risk of development of prostate cancer and to slow its growth, results of human studies are not so clear. Some 15 human epidemiologic studies (studies that examine how various factors affect the occurrence of diseases in population groups) have failed to find a link between the consumption of fish or long-chain, omega-3 fatty acids and the occurrence of prostate cancer. The three notable exceptions include a Swedish study that followed up 6,272 men for 30 years and found that men who ate no fish were two to three times more likely to develop prostate cancer than those who ate moderate or high amounts. More encouragingly, there is considerably stronger evidence, of which we give two examples below, that fish intake can reduce the progression of prostate cancer, resulting in lower rates of locally advanced disease, metastatic disease, and death.

Among 47,882 men participating in the US Health Professionals Follow-up Study who were followed up for 12 years, 2,482 cases of prostate cancer were diagnosed, 617 of which were advanced prostate cancer, including 278 metastatic prostate cancers. Eating fish more than three times per week, compared with less than twice per month, was associated with a reduced risk of prostate cancer, with the strongest association being for metastatic cancer where the risk was reduced by 44 percent. Dark-meat fish had the strongest protective effect, while each additional daily intake of 0.5g of seafood fatty acid was associated with a 24 percent decreased risk of metastatic cancer. Another large study found similar protective effects. The US Physicians' Health Study recruited 20,167 men and followed them up for 19 years, during which time 2,161 cases of prostate cancer developed. Men who consumed fish five times per week or more had a 48 percent lower risk of death from prostate cancer than men who consumed fish less than once per week.

These are not the only studies showing that diet after diagnosis may influence the clinical course of prostate cancer. While there is little evidence for an effect of fish, or fish fatty acids, on the risk of developing prostate cancer, there is a fairly clear indication that fish may offer some protection against disease progression and death from prostate cancer.

How does fish have its effect?
Numerous laboratory and animal studies have consistently shown that fish oils (or long-chain, omega-3 fatty acids) can slow the growth of tumors, prevent their spread, and extend life span. Likely mechanisms include the ability of long-chain, omega-3 fatty acids from fish to compete with long-chain, omega-6 fatty acids (mainly from meat and eggs) for the enzymes that would otherwise convert the omega-6 fatty acids into pro-cancerous products. Increasing the ratio of omega-3 to omega-6 fatty acids in the diet decreased the number of prostate cancer cells in mice, resulting in longer PSA doubling

time. Another important property of fish fatty acids is their ability to prevent the stimulation of growth of prostate-cancer cells by androgens.

Apart from the omega-3 fatty acids, other components of fish, or perhaps the combination, may also be effective against prostate cancer. Seafood is typically high in selenium and oily fish are high in vitamin D, both of which have been linked to protection from prostate cancer.

How much fish do we eat?
Amounts of fish in the diet vary greatly from one part of the world to another, making important contributions to the diets of some coastal communities, but a lesser contribution in landlocked countries. Fish intake in the UK is low, currently about 2 ounces per week per person; given that the average portion is 5 ounces, this is only a third of a portion per week. The most commonly consumed oily fish are salmon, canned or pickled pilchards, sardines, and tuna, canned and smoked mackerel, and fresh trout.

Types of oily fish
Oily fish include kippers, mackerel, pilchards, salmon, trout, herring, sardines, tuna, and anchovies in decreasing order of long-chain, omega-3 fatty acid content. These fish can be fresh, frozen, or canned, with the exception of tuna which loses the beneficial oils when canned.

Other benefits of eating fish
Evidence shows that fish oil can prevent irregular heart rhythm which is probably why it reduces the risk of sudden cardiac death. It also has an

anti-inflammatory effect that may help people suffering from arthritis or other inflammatory conditions. Oily fish may help prevent decline in brain function with age. An additional benefit of fish is that it contains less saturated ("bad") fat than meat. This makes fish a healthier option than meat, not only for prostate health, but also for weight management and heart health. Oily fish also contains vitamin D (see vitamin D section) while all fish are a good source of selenium, vitamin B12, and protein.

Risks of eating oily fish
Pollutants can accumulate in the oils of fish, so no more than four portions of oily fish should be consumed per week. No more than one portion of shark, swordfish, or marlin per week should be consumed, as more pollutants accumulate in the oils of these large predatory fish; pregnant

women and children under the age of sixteen should avoid them. These limits do not apply to non-oily fish. In addition, very large amounts of omega-3s can cause bleeding, but this would require more than one portion per day of the average oily fish.

Recommendations

Given that a protective effect of oily fish is possible, particularly for advanced disease, and that there are other health benefits of eating oily fish, it seems sensible to include it in the diet. In the UK, the recommendations are to consume two portions of fish per week, at least one of which should be oily. This is a minimal, but achievable, amount which may do some good; more would be preferable for optimal effect. Studies have shown benefits at different intakes (see table) but more than two portions per week appear to be required. We recommend two to four portions of oily fish per week, but no more than four because of the pollutants. Other non-oily fish and seafood should also be included in the diet. Note that an average portion is 5 ounces, but can range from about 3½–7 ounces.

Fish

Effects seen at... (according to human studies)	
Fish	2 or more servings per week More than 3 servings per week (metastatic disease) 5 or more servings per week (effects on fatal disease) More than 4½ ounces per day (possible effects at lower amounts)
Fish (mostly oily)	"A large part of the diet" (effects seen at lower amounts)
Fresh or smoked fish	1 or more servings per week
Preserved fish	1–3 servings per month
Target intake...	2–4 portions per week
Good source of...	3½ ounces
Source of...	1½ ounces

legumes, soy, and phytoestrogens

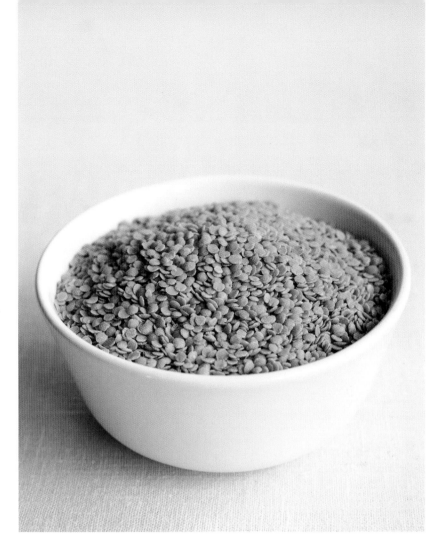

Legumes

Legumes are plants that produce fruit in the form of pods containing edible seeds; the seeds themselves are also known as legumes or pulses. Examples of legumes are peas, beans, lentils, and, surprisingly, peanuts which are often thought of as nuts, although they are in fact legumes. In addition to being excellent sources of protein and fiber, legumes contain many other components that may be beneficial in cancer prevention. Soybeans are among the most commonly consumed legumes, set apart from others by their high content of plant phytochemicals known as phytoestrogens. There is evidence to suggest that both legumes as a whole and soybeans (and soy products) in particular can help fight prostate cancer.

Phytoestrogens are plant compounds that are similar in size and structure to the human hormone estrogen. The term literally means plant (or phyto) estrogen. Numerous classes of phytoestrogens exist, of which one group in particular, the isoflavones, abundant in soybeans, has been most closely linked to prostate cancer prevention. Although isoflavones are present in many legumes, especially fava beans and peanuts, the richest sources are soybeans and their products such

as tofu and soy milk. Diets in many Asian countries are vegetarian and semi-vegetarian, making them rich in plant foods including soy products and therefore phytoestrogens. Given the particularly low rates of prostate cancer in Asian countries, the theory has developed that phytoestrogens are "phytoprotectants" that protect against prostate cancer.

Evidence from human studies

Studies have shown a link between high soy and phytoestrogen intake and a reduced risk of prostate cancer. One study attempted to relate the amounts of a number of different foods consumed in 42 countries to the incidence of prostate cancer. Consumption of a large amount of soy products, including soybeans, was associated with a reduced risk of prostate cancer: in fact soy appeared to be four times more effective than any other food studied. Interestingly men who migrate from Japan, where soy intake is particularly high, to the US, have an increased risk of prostate cancer compared to those who stay in Japan, although, of course, many other factors are likely to be involved as well.

Specific soy foods have been studied in relation to prostate cancer risk. One study investigated the benefit of drinking soy milk: 12,395 men filled out a questionnaire that asked how frequently they used soy milk. Sixteen years later, the number of men who had developed prostate cancer was investigated. Men who drank soy milk once a day appeared to have reduced their risk of prostate cancer by 20 percent, while those who drank soy milk more than once a day reduced their risk by a massive 70 percent. Another prospective study investigated 8,173 Japanese men who had moved to Hawaii, using dietary questionnaires. The men were followed up 19 years later to see who had developed prostate cancer. High tofu (a soy product made from soy milk) intake was found to be linked to a reduced risk of developing the disease and the greater the intake, the stronger was the effect. While other studies have also found protective effects from soy products and soy phytoestrogens, not all have shown such a link.

Consumption of non-soy legumes may also reduce prostate cancer risk as shown in the following three studies. The effect of intake of legumes, both including and excluding soy products, was examined in a study in the US and Canada. Men with prostate cancer (1,619) and men without the disease (1,618) were interviewed about their diet. The researchers found that eating 1½ ounces of soy foods per day reduced the risk of prostate cancer by 38 percent, but eating more than 1³/₄ ounces per day of other legumes reduced the risk by 32 percent. Fourteen thousand men were followed up for six years to examine the effect of diet on prostate cancer risk. The researchers found that eating peas, beans, or lentils more than three times per week, compared to less than once per month reduced the risk of prostate cancer by 47 percent. This can be interpreted as a risk reduction of 18–19 percent with every serving of beans, peas, or lentils per week. In the Netherlands Cohort Study, 58,279 men gave information on their diet at baseline and those who had developed prostate cancer were identified six years later. Eating 2 ounces of legumes per day appeared to reduce the risk of prostate cancer by 29 percent. These studies indicate that legumes in general, not just soybeans, have protective effects against prostate cancer, presumably because of other food components than isoflavones. However, just as for soy foods, not all studies show an effect.

Lignans are another class of phytoestrogens that have been linked to a reduced risk of prostate cancer. Lignans are widely available in the diet but are mainly present in fruits, nuts, and seeds. They are converted by bacteria in the lower gut to the compounds enterolactone and enterodiol which are then absorbed. Though enterolactone has been shown in laboratory studies to reduce cell division and to kill prostate cancer cells, there is only one study linking a lower risk of prostate cancer with higher blood levels of enterolactone.

Though non-soy legumes appear to reduce risk and lignans may be beneficial, it is soy foods for which there is most evidence of an effect.

How do these foods and food components work?
The chemical structure of phytoestrogens allows them to act, weakly, like the human hormone, estrogen, which is essential for both men and women. Isoflavones behave not only as weak estrogens but also as anti-androgens, opposing the activity of testosterone. As these hormones have roles in the development and progression of prostate cancer, it follows that phytoestrogens may have beneficial effects. Testosterone, and the more potent form of testosterone known as dihydrotestosterone (DHT), cause prostate cancer cells to grow. Estrogen can suppress testosterone production. Isoflavones and the compounds they are converted to (their metabolites), such as equol, can act like estrogen to lower testosterone levels, resulting in slower tumor growth. Phytoestrogens can also block the conversion of testosterone into the more potent DHT.

The protective effects of soy foods are thought to be due, at least in part, to their isoflavone content. When soy foods are digested, bacteria living in the gut (large intestine) can metabolize one of the isoflavones (daidzein) into an estrogen-like compound called equol, an antagonist of DHT. Equol can interfere with DHT to reduce its effect and so, reduce prostate cancer risk. However, not everyone has intestinal bacteria that can produce equol, so some people may benefit more from soy foods than others. About 60 percent of vegetarians and 25 percent of non-vegetarians are equol producers. Gut bacteria can also be affected by use of antibiotics and other dietary factors such as the type of carbohydrate.

Furthermore, some 42 percent of northern European men are genetically more able (because of a variation in the estrogen receptor-beta gene) to respond to a high intake of phytoestrogens. A Swedish study showed that these men had an almost 60 percent lower risk of prostate cancer when they had a high (7.3g [¹/₄ ounce] per day) rather than low (0.7g per day) intake of phytoestrogen-rich foods (sum of intake of flaxseed, sunflower seeds, berries, peanuts, beans, and soy). Interestingly, laboratory studies show that phytoestrogens can also act in ways that are unrelated to hormones and these vary according to the type of phytoestrogen. For example, some are weak antioxidants which can help prevent pre-cancerous damage to cells and genes. In laboratories, scientists have shown that isoflavones can halt the growth and cause the death of prostate cancer cells. They can stop the formation of new blood vessels which are required for tumors to grow and they can help prevent a tumor from spreading (metastatic disease). However, it is likely that these particular effects are too weak to be significant in humans. The way non-soy legumes exert their effects may be through the numerous other components present. These include not only some phytoestrogens, but also fiber and a number of other plant chemicals that

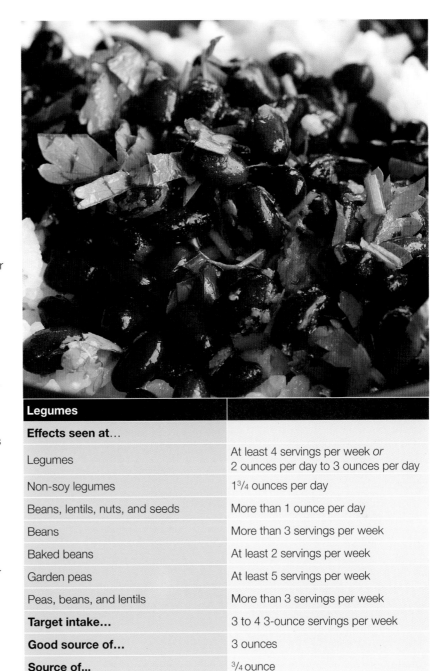

Legumes	
Effects seen at…	
Legumes	At least 4 servings per week *or* 2 ounces per day to 3 ounces per day
Non-soy legumes	1³/₄ ounces per day
Beans, lentils, nuts, and seeds	More than 1 ounce per day
Beans	More than 3 servings per week
Baked beans	At least 2 servings per week
Garden peas	At least 5 servings per week
Peas, beans, and lentils	More than 3 servings per week
Target intake…	3 to 4 3-ounce servings per week
Good source of…	3 ounces
Source of…	³/₄ ounce

Soy and Soy Products

Effects seen at...	
Soybean products	More than 2 servings per week, but even better results at more than one per day
Soy foods	From 1½ to 5¾ ounces per day
Tofu	More than 1 ounce per day *or* More than 5 servings per week *or* 8½ ounces per week
Soy milk	One serving per day, but better effects seen at more than one serving per day (1¾ cups)
Target intake...	3–4 servings of 3 ounces soy food (such as tofu) per week and regular consumption of soy milk
Good source of...	3 ounces soy food or 7 fl. oz. soy milk
Source of...	¾ ounce soy food or 3½ tbsp. soy milk

may work individually, or together, to protect against the disease.

How much of these foods do we eat?

The amounts of soy foods and legumes in people's diets vary greatly worldwide. In the traditional diets of many countries, legumes are combined with cereals (grains). Legumes are also a great source of fiber. They are a dietary staple in some countries of Asia, Latin America, and the Middle East. By contrast, legumes make insignificant contributions to typical North American and most European diets, where meat and other animal foods are eaten in higher amounts.

The legumes consumed in the greatest quantities are soybeans and peanuts. Soybean intake is highest in parts of Asia, and higher than average in parts of Africa and Central America. Intake of isoflavones is correspondingly high in Asian countries such as Japan, where soy food intake is up to 50 times higher than in the UK. Most of the isoflavones in these diets come from the four major soy products, i.e., tofu, miso, natto, and soybean paste.

Sources

The seeds of leguminous plants (legumes) can be eaten as green vegetables, e.g., fava beans and garden peas, and in some cases they are eaten in their pods as is the case for green beans, pole beans, and snow peas. Bean sprouts are legumes that have germinated and sprouted. In some cases, the seeds can mature and dry on the plant, as in lentils and peanuts. Dietary sources of legumes vary across the world; for example, chili beans and refried beans are eaten in Mexico, dal, made from lentils, is eaten in India, pea soup is popular in Sweden, and mung bean sprouts are widely consumed in China.

Soybeans, a rich source of isoflavones, are available dried, frozen, roasted (soy nuts), and fresh (edamame beans). Soybeans are very versatile—see the numerous products listed on page 51. Flaxseed (linseed) is the richest source of lignans though rye (rye bran), cashews, cranberries, and peanuts also contain lignans. Smaller amounts of several types of phytoestrogens are present in a wide variety of fruits, vegetables, legumes, nuts, and seeds, so a variety of such foods may be beneficial.

Other risks and benefits of eating these foods

There has been some concern about the effect of soy foods on thyroid function as soy can reduce the uptake of iodine by the thyroid (i.e., it behaves as a goitrogen). However, a recent review of the evidence found that there was no need to avoid soy foods provided iodine intake was adequate. Those cutting down on milk and dairy products, which are the major sources of iodine in the UK, to less than 2½ cups a day, need to ensure a good alternative source of iodine, such as fish. Non-fish eaters would be well advised to take a supplement that contains iodine (usually a multi-vitamin and mineral supplement). Some questions have also been raised about the safety of soy foods on age-related brain diseases such as Alzheimer's disease. These concerns are based

on one human study which suggested a mild detrimental effect on cognitive (learning and memory) function, but the quality of this study has been questioned and the authors themselves acknowledge that it does not prove a link. Other studies have actually shown benefits of soy foods in relation to brain health. The safety of soy foods has been extensively reviewed and their use is approved by the British Dietetic Association and the US Food and Drug Administration.

Phytoestrogens have been associated with many health benefits including reduced risk of other cancers (e.g., breast cancer), reduced cholesterol levels, blood pressure, heart disease and stroke, improved bone health, and milder menopausal symptoms in women.

Recommendations

We recommend the regular consumption of a variety of legumes. Based on the published evidence, it appears that 3–4 portions per week may be beneficial (3 ounces being one portion). We also recommend an increased intake of soy phytoestrogens (isoflavones) by including soybeans and soy products in the diet. It is difficult to recommend quantities of specific soy foods because the published studies have looked at a variety of soy-containing foods such as soy milk or tofu. However, the data seems to indicate that, again, 3–4 portions of approximately 3 ounces of soy foods per week could have some benefit. Replacing some cow's milk with soy milk would be a simple way to achieve this, in addition to consuming other

soy products. The effects of soy foods were dose-responsive in some studies, meaning that the more that was eaten, the greater the effect. In practical terms, this means that any intake is better than none, even if you cannot meet the target amounts.

The table lists the amounts of legumes and soy foods found to be beneficial in published studies. Our recommendations are derived from this data and our interpretation of the amount that constitutes a "good source of" or "source of" these foods (indicated on the relevant recipes) is shown. It is also advisable to consume a variety of fruits, vegetables, grains, nuts, and seeds (particularly flaxseed and rye) because, although they contain only minimal amounts of phytoestrogens, they will increase overall phytoprotectant intake and form part of a healthy, balanced diet.

Note: a portion of soy foods can constitute a portion of legumes, but a portion of any other legume cannot be considered as a portion of soy, as it will not contain the isoflavones which may be responsible for the beneficial effect of soy.

polyphenols

Thousands of chemicals present in plants are part of a diverse group of plant chemicals known as polyphenols. These give color, odor, and flavor to foods and drinks and have antioxidant and antimicrobial activities which help prevent foods from going off. Many polyphenols are said to have diverse health-protecting qualities, and research indicates that they may slow the growth of human cancers, including prostate cancer. Several polyphenol-rich foods are thought to be beneficial in reducing the risk of prostate cancer but the evidence is strongest for green tea, with growing interest in pomegranate. Some polyphenols—the phytoestrogens, as found in soy foods—are discussed in a separate section.

Green tea has been used for centuries to prevent and treat chronic diseases, and evidence shows it has protective effects against heart disease. The first recorded incidence of tea drinking dates back to 2737 B.C.; now it is the most widely consumed drink in the world, second only to water. Numerous polyphenols are present in tea, accounting for 30 percent of the dry weight of the leaves. Green tea leaves can be fermented to become black tea or partially fermented to become oolong tea. Green tea, in particular, has generated interest in prostate-cancer prevention owing to the low incidence of all types of cancer, including prostate cancer, in

Asian populations where green tea is a popular drink. A growing number of studies supports this association.

Pomegranate is the fruit of a deciduous shrub that has been described as nature's power fruit. It originated in the Middle East but is now grown in the Far East, India, the Mediterranean, and the Americas. A symbol of fertility, life, and healing, the pomegranate has been used for centuries for medicinal purposes, and features in the heraldic crests

of several medical institutions including that of the Royal College of Physicians of London. Components of pomegranate are said to have anti inflammatory, antiatherogenic (reducing build-up of deposits in arteries) and, more recently, anticancer effects.

Evidence from human studies
The results of several studies suggest a protective effect of green tea on prostate cancer. In a much-cited case-control study of men in southeast

China, 130 men with prostate cancer and 274 men without it were asked about their tea-drinking habits (mostly green tea). Analysis showed that green tea-drinkers had a 72 percent lower risk of developing the disease than non-tea-drinkers, and the risk appeared to be reduced with duration, quantity, and frequency of green tea consumption. The best effects were seen with tea drinking over 40 years, consumption of more than $3\frac{1}{3}$ pounds of green tea leaves yearly, and drinking more than four 8 oz. cups daily. The effect was dose-responsive, meaning the greater the intake of tea, the greater the benefit; this means that some tea drinking is better than none at all. In a similar study conducted in Canada on 617 men with prostate cancer and 637 men without it, more than $2\frac{1}{4}$ cups (of 8 oz.) of tea daily was linked to a significantly decreased risk of prostate cancer and the effects were again dose-responsive. It should be noted that the tea consumed was not only green tea.

A prospective study carried out in Japan assessed green-tea consumption in nearly 50,000 men at a certain time point. Fourteen to 17 years later, the number of men who had developed prostate cancer was determined: while analysis showed that green tea had no effect on total prostate cancer, it did reduce the risk of developing advanced disease (cancer that has spread beyond the prostate). The effect was dose-dependent and the greatest effects were seen with consumption of more than five cups (of 8 oz.) per day, which reduced the risk of advanced disease by 47 percent.

An intervention study was carried out in men at high risk of prostate cancer. Thirty men were given a pill containing green tea polyphenols to take every day for a year and 30 men were given a dummy pill (a placebo). After a year, 30 percent of the men in the placebo group (nine men) developed prostate cancer while only 3 percent (one man) developed the disease in those receiving the green-tea pill. This implies that the green-tea pills prevented, or at least delayed, the onset of prostate cancer.

While there are a number of studies to link green tea with cancer-fighting properties, some studies have indicated that even black tea may be protective. The link, however, has not been proved, the evidence is limited and some studies found that tea consumption had no effect. Research in this area is ongoing.

The effects of pomegranate on prostate cancer have been assessed in laboratory and animal studies. These studies have had promising results showing that pomegranate can reduce cell growth and tumor size. However, to date, only one trial has been carried out in humans. In this study, 46 men with rising PSA after surgery or radiotherapy were given a glass (8 fl. oz.) of pomegranate juice per day. Every three months, blood PSA levels were measured. The rise in PSA was significantly slowed down and in seven subjects, PSA levels even dropped. This may indicate a beneficial effect on cancer progression. Importantly, the juice did not cause any adverse effects. The results are promising but do not prove a

link, and other studies are under way to investigate further the potential benefits.

How do polyphenols work?

The anti-cancer effects of green tea are attributed to the many polyphenols present. The most important of these are known collectively as green tea catechins. The mechanisms by which green tea catechins function are interesting as it would seem they have effects against early prostate cancer which is hormone-dependent and also against hormone-independent disease which occurs at a later stage in disease progression.

Androgens stimulate prostate cells to grow and divide, making androgens a target in disease prevention and treatment. In the laboratory, green tea catechins have been found to prevent testosterone from being converted into its more active form, 5-alpha-dihydroxytestosterone, and so may prevent the growth of androgen-sensitive prostate cancer cells. Animal studies have shown that achievable amounts of green-tea polyphenols in the diet reduced the growth not only of androgen-sensitive cells but also of androgen-insensitive cells. These effects were accompanied by increased survival rates. Evidence shows that green tea can kill prostate cancer cells without affecting healthy cells, can delay tumor development, reduce the risk of cancer spread, and even prevent the formation of the new blood vessels required for tumors to grow. The evidence implies that green tea has roles at multiple stages of the disease and so, can be considered not only as a preventive but as a

Albedo

Arils

Outer skin

Membrane

therapeutic agent. Laboratory and animal studies have also shown that green tea may affect the later stages of disease by preventing invasion into surrounding tissues (i.e., metastasis).

Studies carried out in animals have shown that the polyphenols extracted from the juice, peel, and oil of pomegranate may have numerous effects on prostate cancer. These include reported abilities to reduce tumor incidence, delay tumor initiation (the time to getting a tumor), cause prostate cancer cells to die, decrease PSA levels, and slow tumor growth, thereby increasing survival and improving quality of life.

Although this evidence looks promising, there is less evidence for these mechanisms being relevant in humans. The polyphenols may not be absorbed efficiently into the bloodstream and there are questions surrounding, for example, the quantities required, the type of tea,

and the effects in different ethnicities. Other mechanisms, as explained below, may be more important.

Bacteria in the gut, known as gut microflora, play a hugely important role in the effects of polyphenols in the body. The microflora convert the polyphenols into the form in which they appear in the blood, and are delivered to tissues where they can have an effect. For instance, pomegranates contain a class of polyphenols known as ellagitannins and are the only dietary source of galligatannins. These compounds are converted by the gut microflora into urolithins which are probably responsible for the anti-cancer properties ascribed to pomegranates. Due to differences in microflora, some people produce more urolithins than others, so some will benefit more than others from eating pomegranates. Interestingly, it is not only pomegranates that contain ellagitannins; walnuts, berries, particularly raspberries and, to a lesser

extent, strawberries, also contain ellagitannins in smaller amounts and these too are converted to urolithins. It follows that raspberries may also be protective though they have not been studied specifically.

What quantities of polyphenols do we consume?

Two and a three-quarter million tons of dried tea are manufactured annually and consumption varies greatly worldwide. Twenty percent of tea produced is green tea and this is consumed in the highest amounts in Asian countries and a few countries in North Africa and the Middle East. Black tea makes up 78 percent of total tea and is popular in the West and in some Asian countries; the remaining 2 percent is oolong tea, produced and consumed in southeastern China. Tea consumption varies hugely between individuals ranging from no tea to 20 cups per day.

Pomegranate consumption also varies world-wide with production mainly in the Mediterranean and Afghanistan, India, China, Japan, Russia, and some parts of the US. Although the fruit is produced seasonally—typically from September to January in the Northern Hemisphere—the juice is available all year round.

Sources

Polyphenols are widespread in fruits, vegetables, and drinks, but those that have been shown to be particularly relevant to prostate cancer are green tea, pomegranate, and possibly raspberries. Green tea needs to be brewed for five minutes to allow enough time for the active components to be released into the water in sufficient quantities. Black tea, which is made by fermenting green tea leaves, also contains polyphenols and may be benefical in prostate cancer, though the evidence here is weak.

Polyphenols exist in various parts of pomegranate fruit and many exist in the peel. Drinking pomegranate juice may be more beneficial than eating the arils (the seeds surrounded by the little sacs of liquid) as the juice usually includes the peel extract. Pomegranate can be reduced to a syrup, also known as pomegranate paste or pomegranate molasses. This product is used in Middle Eastern cooking and can be bought in specialty Iranian food stores: it can be made at home by reducing the juice in a pan with a little lemon juice and sugar. As noted, ellagitannin polyphenols are also contained in berries, particularly raspberries, although the quantities are not as high as in pomegranate.

There is speculation that a number of other polyphenols have anti-prostate-cancer properties. These include resveratrol in red wine and red grape juice, and curcumin in turmeric, ginger, and cardamom. The research in these areas is in its infancy and so we will have to wait to see whether or not these foods have a noticeable effect.

Other risks and benefits associated with polyphenols
It has been suggested that green tea consumption may benefit many chronic health problems such as inflammatory conditions, diabetes, obesity, cancer, and cardiovascular disease, the latter because of

Green tea	
Effects seen at...	
tea (all types)	More than 2¼ 8-oz. cups per day but less also has an effect
tea (mostly green)	Greater than 4 8-oz. cups per day
green tea	More than 5 8-oz. cups per day but less also has an effect
Target intake...	4–6 cups (8 oz.) per day
Good source of...	1 8-oz. cup

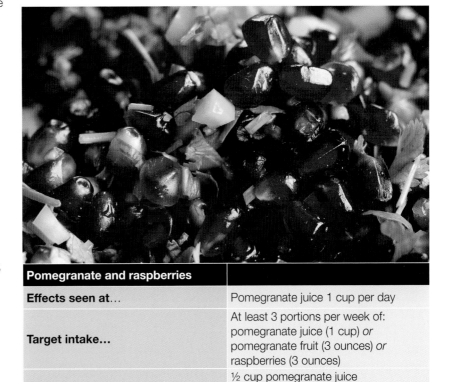

Pomegranate and raspberries	
Effects seen at...	Pomegranate juice 1 cup per day
Target intake...	At least 3 portions per week of: pomegranate juice (1 cup) *or* pomegranate fruit (3 ounces) *or* raspberries (3 ounces)
Good source of...	½ cup pomegranate juice 3 ounces pomegranate fruit 3 ounces raspberries
Source of...	2 tablespoons juice 4 teaspoons pomegranate fruit 2½–3½ tablespoons raspberries

beneficial effects on blood cholesterol. Polyphenols may also improve immune function and have been shown to reduce lower urinary tract symptoms and improve quality of life in men with benign prostate enlargement. An additional benefit of consumption of green tea rather than black tea is that milk and sugar are generally not added.

Fruits such as pomegranate and berries which contain helpful polyphenols are beneficial as part of a healthy, balanced diet in addition to their possible effects on prostate cancer. Pomegranate consumption has been linked not only with reduced risk of prostate cancer but with beneficial effects on the risk of cardiovascular disease.

It is widely accepted that polyphenol-rich foods such as green tea and pomegranate are nontoxic and safe to consume. While green tea is considered safe, the possibility of harmful effects of excessive tea consumption or drinking very hot beverages cannot be ruled out. These risks can be removed by limiting tea intake to no more that six cups per day; this amount has been shown to be beneficial, with benefits also observed at lower levels. This is a conservative limit as intakes in Asia far exceed this amount. Tea could also be left to cool slightly before consumption. The caffeine in green tea may irritate the stomach, cause insomnia or rapid heartbeat, but decaffeinated green tea is available.

There is no evidence of toxicity from pomegranate in humans, even in North Africa where intakes are the highest in the world. Although pomegranate has a long history of use as a food in many cultures, and no studies using pomegranate have found any adverse effects, some people may be allergic to the seeds, so those with known fruit or nut allergies should look out for signs and symptoms of allergic reactions.

Recommendations

As effects of green tea have been seen at quantities of six cups per day, we recommend consumption of four to six cups of green tea per day. This is a safe amount to consume. Effects have been seen at lower doses so any amount would be better than none, even if you cannot reach the ideal six cups. Men taking medication for prostate cancer should not consume more than three cups per day without consulting their physician, as it may potentially slow the rate of drug clearance.

The quantities of polyphenol sources that were effective in studies are shown in the tables on page 29, as well as in our definition of what constitutes a "source" or "good source" in a recipe. In the case of pomegranate and raspberries, it is difficult to recommend a particular amount because only one study of pomegranate has been conducted in humans and no data exist for raspberries. It is likely that long-term regular consumption of pomegranate and raspberries, i.e., roughly three portions per week, would be required for possible benefits.

tomatoes and lycopene

Lycopene is a natural carotenoid pigment that is responsible for the red color of some fruits and vegetables, notably tomatoes. Carotenoids cannot be made in the body and so must be obtained from the diet. In the body, some carotenoids can be converted into vitamin A, while others, including lycopene, act as antioxidants. As lycopene is primarily found in tomatoes, it is this source that is most often studied. However, tomatoes are also an excellent source of other nutrients, including folate, vitamins A, C, and E, potassium, and various other carotenoids and phytochemicals, such as polyphenols, some of which may also be associated with lower cancer risk. It is therefore possible that the anti-cancer effects seen with tomatoes are not due to lycopene alone.

The absorption of lycopene (and other carotenoids) from foods such as tomatoes is helped both by heating and by food processing which help release the lycopene from plant tissues. The addition of a small amount of fat (e.g., olive oil as found in a tomato-based pasta sauce) in which carotenoids are soluble also helps their absorption. Lycopene from fresh watermelon appears to be absorbed well without requiring heating or processing.

Evidence from human studies

According to a number of population studies, men who have a greater dietary intake of either lycopene-containing foods or tomatoes, appear to have a lower risk of developing prostate cancer. When results of 21 such studies were combined, researchers concluded that although tomato products may help prevent prostate cancer, the effect is modest and restricted to those eating large quantities. For instance, men who ate cooked tomatoes or tomato products frequently had a 19 percent reduced risk of getting prostate cancer when compared to those who did not.

In a study of more than 48,000 American health professionals, those who ate two or more portions a week of cooked tomato sauce were 23 percent less likely to develop prostate cancer than those who consumed tomato sauce less than once a month. The same study also reported a decrease in prostate cancer risk, though smaller, for the men with higher intakes of lycopene-containing foods in general.

Twelve small clinical trials have investigated the potential impact of lycopene or tomato consumption on prostate cancer risk or spread. These have mostly been in prostate cancer patients scheduled for prostate removal. Almost all of these trials have found evidence of a good effect on PSA, a marker used for prostate cancer diagnosis and progression (e.g., decreased concentration, decreased velocity, increased stabilization). In one such study in the US, 32 men with localized prostate cancer (awaiting prostate removal) recorded a 20 percent fall in PSA and a 21 percent decrease in DNA damage after three weeks of consuming a daily meal of pasta with tomato sauce containing 30mg of lycopene (approximately 17–18 ounces tomatoes). When compared to a similar but smaller group of prostate cancer patients that had not received the tomato sauce meal, those eating the tomato sauce had 28 percent less damage to their prostate DNA. The amount of lycopene found in the patients' blood had doubled after the three weeks of supplementation while that in the prostate tissue had tripled.

Population studies have suggested ideal levels of lycopene intake ranging from 5–35mg per day. However, it seems that blood levels can be maximized at an intake of 5–10mg lycopene per day. The number of tomato servings shown to have a good effect on prostate cancer risk also varies from as little as three servings per week to over nine, with a beneficial effect from cooked tomato sauce being seen at two or more servings per week.

While these results are encouraging, not all such studies have found an effect on prostate cancer risk with tomato or lycopene consumption. This may be partly due to the known difficulties in measuring food intake accurately, particularly where intakes of lycopene are low. A 2007 US Food and Drug Administration review concluded that currently there was no credible evidence to support a qualified health claim for lycopene, though there was very limited credible evidence for a qualified health claim for tomatoes and/or tomato sauce and a reduced risk of prostate cancer.

How does lycopene work?
Lycopene is the principal carotenoid present in tomatoes, although they also contain significant amounts of two other carotenoids. While lycopene is a highly potent antioxidant, there is limited support for this being its major function in reducing prostate cancer risk. In

Lycopene content in mg per 3½ oz. of food

fact, tissue levels of lycopene appear to be too low for it to play a meaningful antioxidant role. The prostate has levels of the antioxidant alpha-tocopherol (vitamin E) that are 162 times as high as those of lycopene. It now appears more likely that bioactive oxidation products of lycopene, the lycopenoids, are responsible for some of its anti-cancer activity and for the beneficial effects of tomato product consumption. Mechanisms for which there is greater support include induction of death of cancer cells, reduction of damage to DNA, and decreasing androgen levels or activity; for instance, serum testosterone concentrations were significantly decreased in rats that were fed lycopene for four days. It is important to be aware that whole food sources such as tomatoes appear to be more effective than lycopene alone, probably because of the synergism between a number of active food components.

How much lycopene are we getting?
According to the most recent UK National Diet and Nutrition Survey, 67 percent of men between the ages of 19 and 64 consumed raw tomatoes and only 26 percent consumed cooked tomatoes, during the week of the survey. Of those who ate raw tomatoes, the average intake was equivalent to about two tomatoes per week. Of those who ate cooked tomatoes, the average intake was equivalent to only a third of a can of tomatoes per week. There are, of course, other sources of lycopene in the diet that were not taken into account, such as pizza and ketchup.

Other figures on men's tomato consumption come from the EPIC (European Prospective Investigation into Cancer and Nutrition) study and show that the intake of tomatoes and tomato products varies widely across Europe, ranging from 15g per day in the Netherlands to 163g per day in Greece, with an average intake of 64g per day. The average consumption of tomatoes in the US rose considerably at the beginning of the 1990s and leveled off to around ¾ oz. per day for fresh tomatoes (less than two medium-sized tomatoes per week) in 2000. However, the consumption of processed tomato products is much greater in the US and provides the greatest contribution to lycopene intake in the diet there.

Sources of lycopene in the diet
At least 85 percent of the lycopene in our diet comes from tomatoes and tomato products though it is also found in watermelon, pink grapefruit, guava, and rosehip. The lycopene content of tomatoes is variable and increases with ripening, with very red plum tomatoes providing the most. The best sources of lycopene are sun-dried tomatoes, tomato paste, puree and ketchup, as the tomatoes have been concentrated, which gives more lycopene per gram of food. An ideal way of increasing lycopene in your diet is to add an extra tablespoon or two of one of these products to tomato-based dishes that you already cook. These condensed sources, along with canned tomatoes, are a better source of lycopene than raw tomatoes. The chart on the left illustrates the differences in the lycopene content of processed tomato products and raw tomatoes. The table on page 48 details other dietary sources of lycopene.

Other benefits and risks of lycopene

Lycopene may have additional benefits as it has been shown to reduce plasma LDL ("bad") cholesterol and to help reduce the risk of heart attacks, improve immune function, and reduce inflammation. Although lycopene is available in supplement form, those undergoing chemotherapy or radiotherapy should be cautious in taking it in that form as the effect of taking antioxidant supplements during chemotherapy or radiotherapy is unclear. However, the consumption of fruits and vegetables high in antioxidants is believed to be safe during cancer treatment.

Recommendations

As the level of lycopene in the blood (and tissues) reflects dietary intake, foods containing lycopene, particularly tomatoes and tomato products, need to be consumed regularly (strictly speaking, daily, because of the rate of clearance of lycopene) to ensure a continuous supply. We recommend eating meals with a tomato-based sauce at least twice per week. Sources of lycopene other than tomatoes, such as watermelon, have also been used in the recipes to encourage its intake.

The summary table to the right details the quantities of tomatoes consumed in some studies where beneficial effects have been noted, as well as our suggested target intake and our definition of a "good source of" and "a source of" lycopene in the recipes.

Lycopene	
Effects seen at... (according to the study)	3 servings per week to more than 9 servings per week of tomatoes *or* 2 or more servings of cooked tomatoes per week
Target intake...	2 or more servings of cooked tomatoes per week
Good source of...	5mg lycopene
Source of...	1mg lycopene

selenium

Selenium is a trace mineral essential for human health which takes its name from Selene, the Greek goddess of the moon. A number of enzymes that carry out vital functions in the body —including important antioxidant enzymes—rely on selenium for their activity. Lower selenium intakes or levels in body tissues have been linked to higher death rates, greater cancer risk, poor immune function, a reduced ability to deal with viral infections, lower fertility, and age-related brain decline. Research suggests that not only may a higher selenium intake reduce the risk of prostate cancer but, perhaps more importantly, it may be able to suppress the spread of cancer outside the prostate. Many studies have shown that the effect of selenium is even greater in smokers.

Evidence from human trials

The Nutritional Prevention of Cancer (NPC) trial carried out in the Eastern United States provided compelling evidence that selenium could reduce both the risk of developing cancer and the risk of dying from it. A group of 1,312 elderly volunteers, mostly men, were randomly assigned to take either a 200 mcg supplement of selenium yeast or a placebo yeast (dummy tablet) each day for an average period of 4½ years. At the end of 6½ years, the treatment was assessed. In the group that had received selenium rather than the placebo, 37 percent fewer cases of cancer developed

and 50 percent fewer people died of cancer. Most remarkable of all, there were 63 percent fewer cases of prostate cancer. In a follow-up two years later, the effect was slightly less impressive but there were still 49 percent fewer cases of prostate cancer in those that had received selenium.

However, when the differing rates of prostate biopsy in the selenium and placebo groups were taken into account, it appeared that the

only men to benefit from selenium supplementation were those whose PSA was less than 4 when they entered the trial and whose blood selenium was relatively low (i.e., plasma selenium less than 106ng/ml).

A further and much larger American trial—SELECT—did not find any benefit of the same dose of selenium on prostate cancer risk, although a different form of selenium was used. More importantly, SELECT men already had quite high blood levels of selenium (average plasma selenium 135ng/ml) before they joined the trial and, based on the earlier NPC trial results, it could have been predicted that no benefit of giving extra selenium to such men would have been seen.

However, from NPC trial evidence, it would seem that European men, whose blood levels of selenium (average plasma selenium 71ng/ml) are considerably lower than those in the US, could well benefit from increasing their selenium intake. We also now know that because of their genetic make-up, some men need more selenium than others for protection from prostate cancer.

How does selenium work?

The remarkable results of the NPC trial encouraged much research to understand how selenium was having its effect. In fact there is evidence that selenium can act through all the mechanisms shown on pages 9–10. Different mechanisms are likely to come into play at different stages of the disease and according to the type of cancer. Many of the effects of selenium occur through selenoproteins, some of which act as enzymes; amounts of selenium in the diet need to be high enough to make these selenoproteins. Selenium is transported to body tissues by selenoprotein P, which needs a higher selenium intake to optimize it than is usually consumed in Europe. Furthermore, the amount of a specific form of selenium—not a selenoprotein —that has powerful anticancer effects appears to increase as intake goes up. As mentioned above, some people are genetically less able to make the protective selenoproteins, but a higher

dietary intake may help to compensate in such people. In the future it will be possible to tell who is more or less predisposed by a simple genetic test.

How much selenium are we getting?

Selenium enters the food chain through plants, and the amount present in crops varies according to local conditions. Of particular importance is the underlying geology, because it determines the amount and type of selenium present, and the nature of the soil because this affects take-up by the plant.

Because of these factors, intake of selenium varies widely from one part of the world to another as shown in the figure below. In an enormous country like China, it can be both very high in some areas and very low in others. In North America and particularly Canada, intake levels are generally good but in European countries, particularly those of Eastern Europe, intakes are much lower and may be insufficient for the body's requirements.

The amount of selenium in the UK diet and that of many other European countries has declined considerably in recent decades. This is largely due to the fall in imports of selenium-rich strong wheat flour from Canada which was imported for bread making. Other

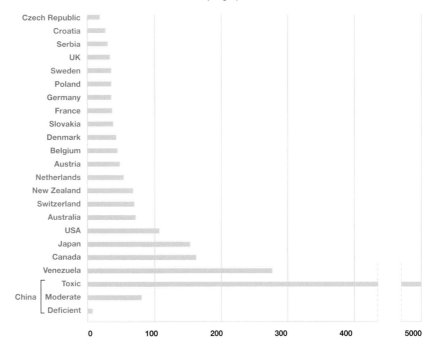

Selenium intake levels (mcg/d) in different countries

factors have also contributed such as breeding cereals for increased grain yield, the fall in acid rain that deposited selenium (along with sulphur), and the increased use of sulphur in fertilizers which competes with selenium for uptake into the plant.

Sources of selenium in the diet

Brazil nuts are the richest natural source of selenium but their selenium content is very variable, ranging from 0.03 to 512mg/g fresh weight. Nuts bought with their shells on appear to contain more selenium than ready-shelled nuts. Brazil nuts also contain a chemical element called barium and the radioactive element radium. Using Brazil nuts as your sole source of selenium is not advisable, as toxic levels of these chemicals could be reached. Organ meats, e.g., liver and particularly kidney, are the next best sources of selenium, followed by fish and seafood. In the UK diet, meat and poultry make the biggest contribution to selenium intake. Game, if eaten, is quite a good source. In countries with high or relatively high selenium intakes (e.g., North America), there will be good levels of selenium in wheat, bread, or other cereals which will therefore make a substantial contribution, but wheat and cereals are not very good sources in most of Europe.

Risk of excessive selenium intake

Selenium, though essential, is toxic in high amounts. The UK Department of Health has set a fairly conservative upper limit of 450mcg per day.

Recommendations

We recommend a target overall consumption of 100–150mcg per day which should be enough to raise the concentration in your blood (and prostate) to levels associated with protective effects. Smokers may wish to aim for the higher end of the range. Good dietary sources of selenium and their selenium content (in mcg/g) are listed on page 48. In the recipes, we have considered 40mcg or more per serving to be a "good source" of selenium and 10–39 mcg per serving to be a "source" of selenium.

Refer to the figure on page 35 to see the level of selenium intake you may already be getting from the typical diet in your country. If the background intake is low, and you do not think you can increase your intake enough from your diet, you may decide to supplement. However, we suggest you supplement with no more than 100mcg per day, preferably as selenium yeast. Remember that your total intake from all sources should *never* exceed 450mcg per day.

vitamin D

Vitamin D is more than just a vitamin, it is also converted to a hormone in the body. It enters the body as the inactive compounds vitamin D3 (cholecalciferol) and vitamin D2 (ergocalciferol) and is converted into the active form $1,25(OH)_2D3$ (calcitriol), as shown in the figure on page 37. The main source of vitamin D3 comes from the action of sunlight on a cholesterol compound in the skin, but it can also be obtained by eating some animal foods such as fish, eggs, and plant foods such as dried shiitake mushrooms. These non-active forms of vitamin D undergo two processes in the body to produce the active form. The first process takes place in the liver where 25(OH)D (calcidiol) is produced. This then circulates in the blood to the kidneys and other tissues where it is converted into the active form, $1,25(OH)_2D$. Blood levels of 25(OH)D can show whether vitamin D status is adequate.

Factors that adversely affect the level of vitamin D in our bodies include lack of exposure to enough sunlight, inadequate intake from diet, and other factors including obesity (vitamin D hides in fat), medication, sunscreen use, skin covered with clothing, skin pigmentation, and age. A 70-year-old produces approximately four times less vitamin D in the skin than a 20-year-old.

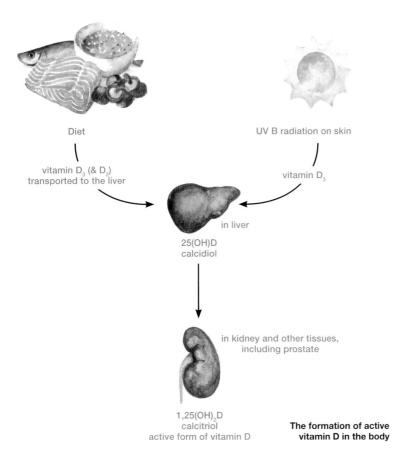

Diet

UV B radiation on skin

vitamin D₃ (& D₂)
transported to the liver

vitamin D₃

in liver

25(OH)D
calcidiol

in kidney and other tissues,
including prostate

1,25(OH)₂D
calcitriol
active form of vitamin D

**The formation of active
vitamin D in the body**

The best-known function of vitamin D is to help us absorb calcium from the diet to build healthy bones. However, we now know that receptors for vitamin D, through which vitamin D interacts, are present in most cells of the body suggesting that vitamin D has other functions.

Evidence from human studies

The "vitamin D-cancer hypothesis" was born when it was observed that people with a history of exposure to high levels of sunlight had a lower risk of a number of cancers. For instance, a significant north–south trend in prostate cancer mortality was found in a 1992 US study, with higher rates in the north where UV radiation was lower. Furthermore, blacks have levels of 25(OH)D that are approximately half those of whites and a 60 percent greater risk of prostate cancer.

However, studies based on blood levels of 25(OH)D or vitamin-D intake do not generally support a link between vitamin D and prostate cancer. The two studies that suggested an increased risk when levels of 25(OH)D were low were conducted in Nordic countries where vitamin D levels get very low in the winter months. In one such study investigating 19,000 Finnish men, those with 25(OH)D levels in the bottom half of the range (below 40 nmol/L) were found to have a 70 percent higher risk of developing prostate cancer than those with levels in the top half. For younger men with 25(OH)D levels in the bottom half, incidence of prostate cancer was 3.5 times higher than for those with levels in the top half, and their incidence of invasive cancer was 6.3 times higher. However, a later study in Nordic populations, while also finding an increased risk at low 25(OH)D levels, found an increased risk in men with the highest values (above 80 nmol/L), suggesting that both low and high vitamin D status could increase risk.

Another strand of evidence for a link between vitamin D and prostate cancer is the fact that men with a particular feature in the DNA that codes for their vitamin D receptor— 14 percent of men of European descent—are more susceptible to this cancer when their blood levels of 25(OH)D are low, and these men also have an increased risk of more aggressive cancer.

As far as we know, there is only one trial of vitamin D in men with prostate cancer: a small Canadian study reported encouraging results in a group of 15 men with recurrent prostate cancer from a daily dose of 50mcg (2000 IU) vitamin D3. PSA levels dropped or stabilized in nine of the men for as long as 21 months, and PSA doubling time increased in 14 men, indicating a reduction in the rate at which PSA levels were increasing.

Taken overall, the evidence for an effect of vitamin D on the risk of developing prostate cancer is confusing. However, the apparent increased risk at high vitamin D levels might be explained by other factors that could be muddying the results. For instance, a high intake of milk, if fortified, will increase vitamin D intake but will also increase calcium intake which can increase the risk of prostate cancer. Vitamin D intake is also associated with vitamin A intake (another fat-soluble vitamin) which may also have antagonistic effects. Another factor that is difficult to account for is obesity which lowers both vitamin D status and PSA.

How does vitamin D work?

$1,25(OH)_2D$ has a number of anti-cancer properties: it causes the death of cancer cells and helps control the process by which they invade surrounding tissue. Directly or indirectly, $1,25(OH)_2D$ controls more than 200 genes, including those responsible for the regulation of cell division, cell death, and the creation of new blood vessels without which a cancer cannot grow.

Many cells, including prostate cells, contain the enzyme that is responsible for the conversion of $25(OH)D$ to $1,25(OH)_2D$ so they can produce active vitamin D independently of the kidneys. Low levels of circulating $1,25(OH)_2D$ have been associated with an increased risk of aggressive disease. Unfortunately, when prostate cells become cancerous, they appear to lose the ability to produce $1,25(OH)_2D$. For that reason, the important time to have good vitamin D status may be many years before the cancer develops.

How much vitamin D are we getting?

Most of the vitamin D (90 percent) in our bodies is made in the skin following exposure to sunlight. Above latitude 37° in the Northern hemisphere, from November to February, there is not enough sunlight of the right wavelength to produce vitamin D (the same applies below 37° in the Southern hemisphere). The time of day is also important; for instance in the UK, at 54° of latitude, the appropriate wavelength of sunlight is only available between 11am and 3pm from March through to October. Cloud cover also inhibits vitamin D production, as does pollution, sunscreen, enveloping clothing, elderly and dark skin. People with dark skins produce no more than 5–19 percent of the vitamin D produced in light-skinned people. Intake from diet is therefore much more important in such people and at northern latitudes, particularly in the winter.

The level of $25(OH)D$ measured in blood serum shows the extent of deficiency. Many scientists think the level should be approximately 75nmol/L (30ng/ml) to provide optimal health protection. However, with the exception of Norway, where vitamin D-rich oily fish consumption is relatively high, vitamin D status in Europe in winter does not reach such levels. A recent investigation showed that low vitamin D status was widespread in white British adults aged 45, with 87 percent having levels of $25(OH)D$ during the winter/spring below the 75nmol/L thought to be required for optimal

bone health, and 47 percent having levels low enough to warrant vitamin D supplementation. A UK study of over-65-year-olds showed that 8 percent had blood concentrations of $25(OH)D$ lower than the minimum 25nmol/L needed to prevent rickets and softening of the bones, while 97 percent were not consuming the minimum recommended level of 10mcg/d vitamin D from food. Intakes in Germany and the Netherlands are almost as low as in the UK, though slightly higher in Finland where more oily fish is consumed.

Current guidelines on vitamin D intake

For UK adults under the age of 65 years, there is no recommended intake level for vitamin D. For those over this age or at risk of deficiency, the suggested intake is 10mcg per day. However this level is set to prevent the onset of osteomalacia (softening of the bones), and does not take into account the additional roles of vitamin D. The adequate intakes suggested in the US are 5mcg per day for adults aged 19–50, 10mcg for adults aged 51–70 years, and 15mcg for those over 70. However, many scientists believe these guidelines to be too low.

Food sources of vitamin D

Very few foods naturally contain vitamin D. Oily fish are the best sources. Fortified cereals, margarine, and most reduced- or low-fat spreads are also an important source due to the regularity with which they are consumed. Foods such as milk and orange juice are fortified in some countries including the US, resulting in a higher vitamin D intake. The table on page 48 shows food sources of vitamin D.

Risk of excessive vitamin D intake

Excessive intake of vitamin D can promote excessive levels of calcium in the blood. However, vitamin D doses up to 25mcg (1000 IU) per day appear to have no associated toxicity and this is the safe upper level that has been set by the UK Expert Group on Vitamins and Minerals for supplementary vitamin D intake. The EU Scientific Committee on Food Opinion and the US Standing Committee on the Scientific Evaluation of Dietary Reference Intakes have set a higher safe intake, 50mcg (2000 IU) per day. However, remember as discussed above, that some studies have found an increased risk of prostate cancer, particularly of aggressive prostate cancer, in men with higher vitamin D status.

Other benefits of vitamin D

In addition to its classical function in bone health, there is good evidence for a benefit of vitamin D in prevention of colorectal cancer. Furthermore, combined results from 18 trials showed that vitamin D supplements (10–20 mcg/400-800 IU, per day) lowered the risk of death from all causes in people over 50 years old, many of whom had low vitamin D status to start with, though only by a modest amount i.e., 7 percent. Additional effects have been described in the regulation of the immune system (e.g., in autoimmune diseases such as multiple sclerosis and rheumatoid arthritis), blood pressure, congestive heart failure, chronic kidney disease, muscle function, and an improvement in type II diabetes.

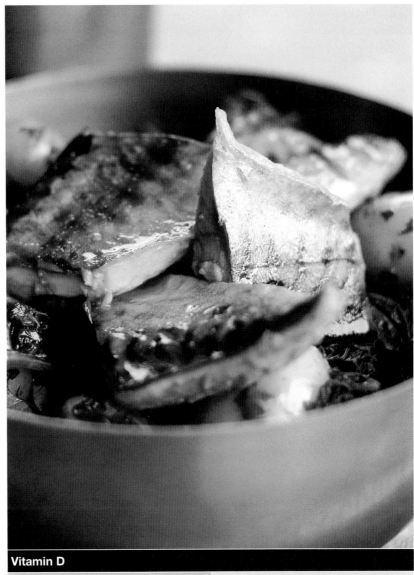

Vitamin D	
Target intake...	2–4 portions of oily fish per week plus other dietary sources of vitamin D (see table on page 48)
Good source of...	8mcg
Source of...	2mcg

Recommendations

Although the evidence linking vitamin D to a reduced risk of prostate cancer is weak and only seems to apply to men with vitamin D deficiency (less than 40 nmol/L), a certain amount of vitamin D is essential for good health. Many people with dark skin, and/or living in northern latitudes have deficient vitamin D status, which can be improved through diet. If you fall into these categories, we recommend the intake of two to four portions of oily fish per week, and the regular consumption of foods fortified with vitamin D (margarine, fortified breakfast cereals, and fortified milk and orange juice in the US). If you do not think you can achieve this intake from diet, you may wish to consider supplementing, particularly in the winter when you have no sun exposure, but we recommend that you should not go above current US guidelines of 10–15mcg per day and on no account should you exceed 25mcg (1,000 IU) per day.

The summary table on page 39 details our suggested target intake and our definition of a "good source of" and "a source of" that has been included in the recipes.

vitamin E

Vitamin E is the collective term for a group of eight similar chemicals made by plants. Vitamin E is essential for human health and has important antioxidant roles as well as apparently beneficial effects on the risk of various disorders such as atherosclerosis, heart disease, and cancer. Of the eight forms of vitamin E, alpha-tocopherol (the form found in supplements) is by far the most biologically active, while gamma-tocopherol has other important protective functions. Though inconsistent and limited, there is evidence to suggest that vitamin E may have a protective role in prostate cancer development and progression.

Evidence from human studies

A number of studies have assessed the effects of vitamin E on prostate cancer risk. Some assessed vitamin E intake from diet or supplements while others measured the amount of vitamin E circulating in the blood. Findings have varied with some studies showing a benefit associated with higher levels of vitamin E intake or blood levels, and others showing no effect. Most studies that assessed vitamin E intake found that supplements, rather than high intakes from food alone, appeared to have the greatest effect. It was noticeable that the benefits were stronger in smokers than in non-smokers, and for advanced prostate cancer rather than total prostate cancer. The studies that assessed blood levels

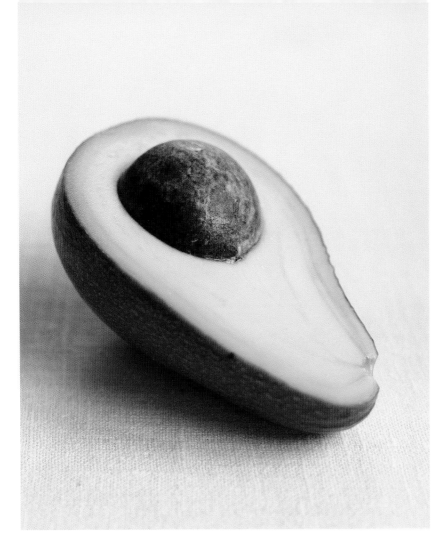

of vitamin E were more inconsistent in their findings but again indicated that smokers may gain more benefit than non-smokers. Interestingly, one study showed that gamma-tocopherol appeared to have more benefit than alpha-tocopherol.

The strongest evidence for a protective effect of vitamin E on prostate cancer risk comes from the ATBC (Alpha-Tocopherol Beta-Carotene) trial carried out in Finland and published in 1998.

In the trial, 29,133 male smokers were given supplements of either alpha-tocopherol (50mg or 75 IU), beta carotene, neither, or both for approximately six years to test their effect on lung-cancer risk. In the group that took the alpha-tocopherol supplements, there were 32 percent fewer prostate cancer cases and 41 percent fewer deaths from prostate cancer. Notably, the supplements appeared to protect from the spread of tumors beyond the prostate gland. By contrast, the US Physicians'

Health Study, published in December 2008, found no effect of supplements of synthetic alpha-tocopherol (267mg [400IU] on alternate days) or vitamin C (500mg per day) on prostate-cancer risk. However, a major difference between the two studies was the very small number of participants who smoked, so if the beneficial effect of vitamin E is predominantly in smokers, according to the authors, it would likely have been missed in that trial.

How does vitamin E work?

Vitamin E is best known for its antioxidant activities which enable it to protect cells and DNA from damage. Vitamin E has been shown to inhibit the growth of various types of cells, to reduce tumor growth in mice, to cause prostate cancer cells to die, and to reduce levels of testosterone, a hormone which is required for the growth of prostate cancer cells. Although alpha-tocopherol is generally considered the most potent form of vitamin E, gamma-tocopherol has unique protective effects including reduction of inflammation, suggesting that it may potentially be more important in protection from prostate cancer.

Vitamin E intake

While alpha-tocopherol is the usual form in supplements and in European diets, gamma-tocopherol is quantitatively the largest vitamin E component in the US diet. It should be noted that high doses of alpha-tocopherol reduce the level of blood and tissue gamma-tocopherol, a potentially undesirable effect.

Sources

Vitamin E is made by plants and is fat-soluble; this means that it is found predominantly in the fats and oils of plants. Good sources of vitamin E include wheat germ, vegetable oils and margarine, nuts and nut oils, seeds such as sunflower seeds and some legumes including soybeans and chickpeas (see table on page 48). Other good sources include egg yolk, Parmesan and cheddar cheese, oatmeal, olives, avocados, carrots, green leafy vegetables, sweet potatoes, tomatoes, and watercress. In addition, some cereals are fortified with vitamin E. Fat spreads, cereals, and cereal products make important contributions to vitamin E intakes in the UK.

Other benefits of vitamin E

Vitamin E may have protective effects against cancers in other sites including esophageal (gullet), gastric, lung, and colorectal cancers. It is also thought to reduce the risk of atherosclerosis and heart disease, partly because it can limit the oxidation of fats in the body.

Risk of excessive vitamin E intake

Levels of vitamin E up to 1,000mg (1500 IU) per day can normally be tolerated without causing harm, although increased blood-clotting times have been seen above 400mg (600 IU) per day in some people. This effect on clotting time may explain the increased risk of hemorrhagic stroke seen in some studies where vitamin E supplements were given. Long-term use of 268mg (400 IU) vitamin E supplements by patients with diabetes or poor blood flow through the arteries was linked to increased risk of heart failure and death. Supplementation with high dosages of vitamin E could also interfere with medicinal drugs, potentially reducing the benefits of drug therapy.

Recommendations

While some studies indicate a protective role of vitamin E, in general findings are inconsistent and far from conclusive. The evidence of a beneficial effect of vitamin E is strongest for smokers and at supplemental levels, rather than from high intakes from food alone. An additional intake of as little as 10mg per day is likely to be enough to raise the concentration of vitamin E in the blood to a level associated with protection. Changing diet can be effective as shown by a study in which people were put on a diet rich in rapeseed oil (canola oil), a readily available and inexpensive cooking oil that is a good source of gamma-tocopherol. At the end of three weeks, their blood levels of gamma-tocopherol had increased by 23 percent, while those of alpha-tocopherol had risen by 7 percent.

We recommend trying to increase intake of vitamin E through dietary means. Smokers may want to consider vitamin E supplements but they would be well advised to look for a low-dose supplement, ideally no more than 50mg (75 IU) per day (as in the ATBC trial). Given the time for vitamin E to be cleared from the system, it would probably be equally good to take a 100mg supplement (which may be easier to find) every other day. Try to find a vitamin E supplement that contains mixed tocopherols which will contain gamma-tocopherol as well. Those on medication should consult their doctor before supplementing and should not go above a dose of 134mg (200 IU) per day.

None of the recipes here will be termed a "good source" because few foods contain particularly high amounts of vitamin E and those that do are high in fat, which would increase the calorie and fat content of the recipe if large amounts were to be used. We have termed recipes that contain 3mg or more per serving a "source of" vitamin E, as this is a relatively high amount to have in one meal.

foods to consume in limited amounts

Inevitably, when research is carried out into the links between diet and prostate cancer, some foods or food components will show a positive relationship, meaning that eating them in large amounts may actually increase the risk of prostate cancer. The foods that have been suggested as having a "positive relationship" include dairy products, fat, and meat.

dairy products

Dairy products include milk and all products made from milk, such as yogurt, cheese, and fromage frais. The evidence for an association between prostate cancer and dairy products comes from population studies. Although most studies seem to show an association with increased risk of prostate cancer, there are some that show no association or even a decreased risk, although these have mainly been carried out on population groups with moderate or low intake of dairy foods. The explanations for the proposed increased risk of prostate cancer from dairy products have generally focused on their content of calcium and phytanic acid.

Calcium

Dairy products provide our main source of calcium, and some studies have shown a relationship between high intakes of calcium and increased prostate cancer risk. One of the reasons suggested for this increased risk is the relationship between calcium and vitamin D, a potential anti-cancer agent. Calcium requires the action of vitamin D to aid its absorption. Therefore, when calcium intakes are high, the demand for vitamin D increases and may lead to the suppression of vitamin D in the blood.

The relationship between an increased risk of prostate cancer and calcium appears to be most apparent when calcium intake is very high (1,500–2,000mg per day) and in cases where the disease is more advanced, although the evidence is not consistent. Interestingly, studies that have considered the risk of prostate cancer with non-dairy sources of calcium appear to show no association, although the effect of calcium supplementation is unclear.

Phytanic acid

Phytanic acid is a fatty acid found in dairy products and in ruminant animal meat such as beef and lamb. A small study showed that the amount of phytanic acid in the blood of prostate cancer patients was higher than that in the blood of people without prostate cancer. This same study also showed that the blood levels of phytanic acid in this group of people were related to the amounts of dairy foods and red meat in their diets. A role for phytanic acid in the development and progression of prostate cancer was therefore suggested.

The effect of phytanic acid on prostate cancer risk has also been linked to the over-expression of a gene in prostate cancer cells that is responsible for the breakdown of phytanic acid. This has led to speculation that prostate-cancer cells may use this fatty acid as an energy source which can help them to grow.

Current guidelines for the consumption of dairy foods

Dairy foods represent a major food group that is widely consumed and encouraged as part of a healthy balanced diet. Healthy eating guidelines (the UK "Eatwell Plate" and the US "MyPyramid" food pyramid) recommend that dairy foods should make up about one sixth of the food eaten by adults each day in the UK, or one fifth of the food eaten by adults each day in the US. This equates to 568ml (about 2½ cups) or 732ml (three cups) of milk, or the equivalent in a combination of dairy foods, such as 189–244ml (¾–1 cup) of milk, plus 120g or 1–½ cup (245g) of yogurt and 1–1½ ounces of cheese. This intake would provide between 700 and 1,000mg of calcium per day which meets the recommended calcium intake for the adult population in many countries, and provides most of the recommended intake in the countries that have set a higher target.

Recommendations

The current guidelines for the consumption of dairy foods should not increase the risk of prostate cancer. However, the evidence does seem to suggest a possible association with high intakes. Therefore those who regularly consume quantities greater than the recommended intakes should consider substituting some of their intake with non-dairy alternatives such as soy products (not calcium-fortified) which have been suggested as having a beneficial effect on prostate cancer. While dairy products provide one of the best sources of calcium, there are a number of other good dietary sources including dark-green leafy vegetables such as spinach and kale, oily fish with bones such as sardines, and dried apricots, all of which can be included in a healthy and varied diet.

If a decision is made to undertake a dairy-free diet, it should only be done with advice from a qualified dietitian. Dairy products are a major source of calcium and iodine, and supplementation should be considered if they are not supplied in sufficient quantities in the diet. Calcium is essential for bone health which could be compromised in men receiving hormone therapy, resulting in a greater risk of osteoporosis (softening of the bones). It is therefore important that these men follow the advice of their doctor regarding the prescription of calcium supplements.

Considering the possible association of high intakes of dairy foods with prostate cancer, the majority of the recipes in this book are dairy-free, contain only a little dairy, or give options for the inclusion of dairy-free alternatives. Where possible, the dairy component of the recipe is replaced with soy to provide more of the beneficial ingredients.

fat

A high intake of fat has been identified as a key contributor to non-communicable diseases such as heart disease. Its relationship with prostate cancer also appears to be a detrimental one. In countries where fat intake is relatively low, there appears to be a low incidence of prostate cancer. Research has generally supported the association between high intakes of fat, particularly saturated or animal fats, and increased risk of prostate cancer, across a range of ethnic groups. Diets high in fat are also likely to be high in calories, thereby promoting obesity which is associated with more aggressive prostate cancer and prostate cancer mortality. Encouragingly, some studies have suggested that low-fat diets may slow the progression of prostate cancer, particularly to the hormone-independent stage. While the general message is to choose low-fat foods, especially those low in saturated or animal fats, there are some high-fat foods, such as oily fish, that are probably beneficial and should be included in a diet aimed at prostate health.

Effects of different types of fat
Dietary fat can be divided into different types of fatty acids including saturated fatty acids, monounsaturated fatty acids (MUFA), and polyunsaturated fatty acids (PUFA). The PUFA group has further sub-groups, the omega-6 and omega-3 fatty acids.

The omega-3 fatty acid group includes the long-chain PUFAs from fish oils that appear to offer some protection against prostate-cancer progression and death (see Fish section). Alpha-linolenic acid is an omega-3 fatty acid of plant origin that has been suggested to be detrimental to prostate cancer risk. In the US, important sources of alpha-linolenic acid are margarine, butter, mayonnaise, oil- and vinegar-based and creamy salad dressings, and beef, pork, and lamb. However, some studies have shown no association with alpha-linolenic acid or even a decreased risk.

Diets high in omega-6 fatty acids may promote the growth of cancer cells, probably because they are converted to inflammatory compounds that can stimulate tumor growth. Linoleic acid, which is found in most vegetable oils and margarines, is the most common omega-6 PUFA in the Western diet, accounting for 8.9 percent of energy intake (compared to 0.8 percent in the Far East), and makes a significant contribution to total fat intake.

There is some suggestion that intake of MUFA, found in foods such as olive oil, rapeseed oil (canola oil), and avocados, is associated with an increase in prostate cancer risk, although when olive oil is looked at specifically, the effect appears to be protective, perhaps because olive oil has other beneficial components. Saturated fatty acids which are predominantly from animal sources, such as the fat on meat, appear to be the fatty acid group most associated with an increase in prostate cancer risk.

Although the mechanisms linking fat and its various components to prostate cancer risk are unclear, effects on testosterone levels, insulin-like growth-factor-1 (a promoter of prostate cancer growth), and inflammation, a factor known to contribute to prostate cancer risk, may well be involved.

Recommendations

As the evidence relating to a detrimental effect of specific fatty acids is unclear, the current recommendations for fat intake which are also beneficial for heart health provide the most appropriate guideline for prostate health. Total fat intake should constitute no more than 25–35 percent of total energy intake, with saturated fat being limited to 10 percent of total energy intake. Ways to help achieve this include choosing lean cuts of meat, removing any excess fat, removing the skin from poultry, as well as choosing oils and spreads that are higher in polyunsaturated fatty acids and particularly omega-3 fatty acids and monounsaturated fatty acids such as olive oil. For instance, you could replace butter with olive spread or an omega-3 spread, use canola oil for frying and olive oil for salads. By making these changes, you will not only be reducing the intake of saturated fat but also the intake of omega-6 fatty acids, which are associated with undesirable inflammatory effects.

meat

There is some evidence that diets high in meat, particularly red and processed meats, may increase the risk of prostate cancer. In a 2001 review of 22 studies, 16 of them showed a 30 percent or more increased risk associated with meat intake. By contrast, the 2007 World Cancer Research Fund/American Institute for Cancer Research (WCRF/AICR) review of diet and cancer found that no conclusions could be drawn on the relationship between prostate-cancer risk and meat in general, though there was some evidence to support an increase in risk from eating processed meat.

Because results are inconsistent, it has been suggested that other dietary components associated with meat may be possible promoters or inhibitors of risk. For instance, meat intake has also been associated with high fat intake which, as we have discussed, may also have cancer-promoting effects. Furthermore, diets high in meat may also be low in protective fruits and vegetables. Ruminant meats, such as beef and lamb, are also a source of phytanic acid, which has been linked to an increase in the risk of prostate cancer in the case of dairy produce. Red meat is a major source of zinc which promotes testosterone synthesis. Perhaps more importantly, the way in which meat is often cooked can lead to the formation of undesirable cancer-causing compounds.

A number of studies have compared the relationship between the degree of meat cooking and prostate cancer risk. Meat that is "well done" and "very well done" is more likely to increase the risk of prostate cancer. When muscle meats are cooked at high temperatures, a group of substances known as heterocyclic amines can be formed. Heterocyclic amines have been listed as substances "reasonably anticipated to be human carcinogens" by the US Department of Health and Human Services. Other cooked animal foods such as eggs, milk and organ meats (e.g., liver and kidney) contain only very small amounts of heterocyclic amines. Furthermore, cooking on charcoal grills can deposit polycyclic hydrocarbons, which are known to cause cancer, on the outside of the meat.

Recommendations

To help prevent and control cancers, the WCRF/AICR recommend consuming less than 18 ounces per week of red meat, only a little of which should be processed meat. While this is a reasonable target, it is important to note that meat is part of a valuable food group that provides protein to build and repair body tissues, as well as many essential vitamins and minerals, such as iron. There are of course other sources of protein such as fish, eggs, soy, and legumes that can substitute for some meat. If a decision is made to remove meat from the diet completely, it should be done only after careful consideration of the nutritional content of the diet as a whole, and ideally with the advice of a dietitian.

The US National Cancer Institute (NCI) offers the following advice to reduce the formation of heterocyclic amines when cooking meat: "Concerned individuals can reduce their exposure to heterocyclic amines by varying methods of cooking meats; microwaving meats more often, especially before frying, broiling, or barbecuing; and refraining from making gravy from meat drippings." In line with these recommendations, we have for the most part included recipes where meat is cooked in a sauce to try to limit the formation of heterocyclic amines, and no meat is barbecued. Furthermore, a number of the recipes have used reduced serving sizes of meat or suggest how this may be achieved.

Foods to consume in limited amounts – examples

Dairy Products	Saturated Fat	Red and Processed Meat*
Cheese	Cookies	Beef
Cheese sauce	Butter	Pork
Cheesecake	Cakes	Lamb
Condensed milk	Coconut cream	Goat
Cream	Coconut oil	Bacon
Crème caramel	Cream	Hot dogs
Crème fraîche	Crème fraîche	Ham
Custard	Dried coconut	Hamburgers
Dried milk	Ghee	Pastrami
Evaporated milk	Hard cheese	Salami
Flavored milk	Lard	Sausages
Fromage frais	Meat fat	
Ice cream	Meat pies	* defined by WCRF/ AICR 2007
Milk	Meat products	
Milkshake	Palm oil	
Mousse	Pastry	
Rice pudding	Salami	
Semolina	Sausages	
Sour cream	Sour cream	
Tzatziki		
White sauce		
Yogurt		

Suggested intakes for dairy foods, dietary fat, and meat

Dairy foods...	No more than 2½ cups or 3 cups of milk or the equivalent in dairy foods (see page 44 for more details)
Dietary fat...	Total fat should not be more than 25–35 percent of total energy intake Saturated fat should not be more than 10 percent of total energy intake
Meat...	No more than 18 ounces per week of red meat, to include only a little processed meat Avoid burnt meat, and cooking meat at high temperatures, e.g., barbecuing

Sources of the foods and food components beneficial for prostate cancer

Food	Amount per 100 g	Portion size (g)	Amount per portion
Lycopene			
Tomato juice	9.0 mg	160	14.4 mg
Tomato soup	5.3 mg	220	11.7 mg
Watermelon	4.5 mg	200 (large slice)	9.0 mg
Tomato paste	28.8 mg	15 (1 tbsp)	4.3 mg
Tomato puree	21.8 mg	15 (1 tbsp)	3.3 mg
Tomato ketchup	15.2 mg	20	3.0 mg
Guava	5.4 mg	55	3.0 mg
Papaya	2.0–5.3 mg	140 (average slice)	2.8–7.4 mg
Canned tomatoes	2.8 mg	100	2.8 mg
Tomatoes (raw)	2.6 mg	85 (1 medium)	2.2 mg
Pink grapefruit	1.4 mg	125 (½ medium)	1.8 mg
Sundried tomatoes	45.9 mg	2 (1 piece)	0.9 mg
Baked beans	0.5 mg	135	0.7 mg
Dried apricots	0.9 mg	40g (5 apricots)	0.4 mg
Vitamin E			
Sunflower seeds	37.8 mg	16 (1 tbsp)	6.0 mg
Salmon	3.9 mg	100	3.9 mg
Pecans	26.7 mg	14 (10 halves)	3.8 mg
Almonds	24.0 mg	13 (6 whole)	3.1 mg
Sardines (tinned in tomato sauce)	3.1 mg	90	2.8 mg
Sweet potato	4.6 mg	65 (1 medium)	3.0 mg
Hazelnuts	25.0 mg	10 (10 whole)	2.5 mg
Avocado	3.2 mg	75 (½ pear)	2.4 mg
Canned tuna (in oil)	1.9 mg	92	1.8 mg
Brazil nuts	14.4 mg	12 (3 nuts)	1.7 mg
Sunflower oil	49.2 mg	3 (1 tsp)	1.5 mg
Spinach	1.7 mg	90	1.5 mg
Peanuts	10.1 mg	13 (10 whole)	1.3 mg
Wheat germ	22.0 mg	5 (1 tbsp)	1.1 mg
Palm oil	33.1 mg	3 (1 tsp)	1.0 mg
Tomatoes	1.2 mg	85 (I medium)	1.0 mg
Walnuts	3.9 mg	20 (6 halves)	0.8 mg
Margarine	7.9 mg	10 (on slice of bread)	0.8 mg
Eggs	1.1 mg	61 (I size 2)	0.7 mg
Soybean oil	18.2 mg	3 (1 tsp)	0.6 mg
Peanut oil	15.6 mg	3 (1 tsp)	0.5 mg
Mango	1.1 mg	40 (1 slice)	0.4 mg
Pine nuts	11.2 mg	1.7 (10 nuts)	0.4 mg
Sesame seeds	2.5 mg	12 (1 tbsp)	0.3 mg
Olive oil	5.1 mg	3 (1 tsp)	0.2 mg

Food	Amount per 100 g	Portion size (g)	Amount per portion
Vitamin D			
Herring	16.1 mcg	119	19.2 mcg
Trout	9.6 mcg	155	14.9 mcg
Mackerel	8.8 mcg	160	14.1 mcg
Pilchards (canned in tomato sauce)	14.0 mcg	100	14.0 mcg
Salmon	7.1 mcg	100	7.1 mcg
Sardines (tinned in tomato sauce)	8.0 mcg	100	8.0 mcg
Shiitake mushrooms (sun-dried)	41.5 mcg	10	4.2 mcg
Tuna (canned in oil)	3.0 mcg	92	2.8 mcg
Eggs	1.8 mcg	61 (I size 2)	1.1 mcg
Margarine	7.9 mcg	10 (on slice of bread)	0.8 mcg
Fortified breakfast cereals	2.8–8.3 mcg	30	0.8–2.5 mcg
Butter	0.9 mcg	10 (on slice of bread)	0.1 mcg
Selenium			
Kidney lamb/pig	150 mcg	112	168 mcg
Brazil nuts (NB very variable content)	1530 mcg	12 (3 nuts)	153 mcg
Lemon sole	60 mcg	170	102 mcg
Tuna (canned in oil)	90 mcg	92	83 mcg
Swordfish	45 mcg	140	63 mcg
Lobster	41 mcg	150	62 mcg
Mackerel	30 mcg	160	48 mcg
Liver (lamb)	42 mcg	100	42 mcg
Sardines (canned)	41 mcg	100	41 mcg
Pork	34 mcg	120	40 mcg
Crab	37 mcg	85	32 mcg
Sardines (fresh)	34 mcg	86 (6 sardines)	29 mcg
Chicken	12 mcg	150	18 mcg
Duck	12 mcg	150	18 mcg
Pheasant	16 mcg	110	17 mcg
Turkey (light meat)	10 mcg	150	15 mcg
Shrimp	16 mcg	60	10 mcg
Eggs	11 mcg	61	7 mcg
Cashews	20 mcg	20	4 mcg

These figures are taken from the United States Department of Agriculture, McCance and Widdowson's 'The Composition of Foods' and a number of scientific studies.

Sources of the foods and food components beneficial for prostate cancer

Allium Vegetables
Chives
Garlic
Leeks
Onion
Scallions (spring onions)
Shallots

Cruciferous Vegetables
Bok choy (Pak choi)
Broccoli
Brussels sprouts
Cabbage
Cauliflower
Garden cress
Horseradish
Kale
Mustard
Radish
Arugula (rocket)
Rutabaga (swede)
Wasabi
Watercress

Oily fish
Anchovies
Bloater (like larger kippers)
Carp
Eel
Herring
Kippers
Mackerel
Pilchards (large sardines)
Salmon
Sardines
Brisling
Swordfish
Trout
Tuna
Whitebait (a variety of smelt)

Phytoestrogens
Soy
Meat alternatives, e.g., soy bacon, sausages, and burgers
Miso soup
Natto (an Asian food)
Soybeans (edamame, available frozen or dried)
Soy cereal
Soy cheese
Soy custard
Soy dip
Soy flour
Soy ice cream
Soy and linseed bread
Soy milk
Soy nuts (roasted soybeans)
Soy pasta
Soy protein
Soy sauce
Soy spread
Soy yogurt
Tempeh (an Asian food)
Tofu (soybean curd)

Legumes
Beans, e.g., fava, black, navy (haricot), white, pinto, kidney, aduki
Chickpeas
Lentils
Peanuts
Peas

Lignans
Cashews
Cranberries
Flaxseed (linseed)
Peanuts
Raisins
Rye (bran)

Polyphenols
Green tea
Pomegranate fruit
Pomegranate juice
Raspberries
Strawberries

breakfasts

blueberry smoothie

This smoothie is easy to prepare and makes a refreshing start to the day. A bonus is that blueberries boost your concentration.

SERVES 2

- 1 cup blueberries
- 1 cup raspberry-flavored soy yogurt
- soy or rice milk, for diluting

Put the blueberries and yogurt in a blender and blend until smooth.

Blend in enough milk to reach the desired consistency.

Good source of soy. Source of vitamin E
PER PORTION: 148 CAL, 3.6G FAT, 0.7G SATURATED FAT

pomegranate and guava smoothie

This smoothie makes a great snack at any time of the day.

SERVES 2

- 1 14-oz. can guavas, drained and seeded
- 1 medium ripe banana
- 1¼ cups pomegranate juice, plus extra to loosen

Put the fruit and juice in a blender and blend until smooth.

Blend in a little extra pomegranate juice to reach the desired consistency.

Good source of polyphenols. Source of lycopene
PER PORTION: 221 CAL, 0.2G FAT, 0.1G SATURATED FAT

oatmeal with raspberry and pomegranate compote

This is a warming breakfast that is quick to make. The compote can be made a day or so in advance and refrigerated until ready to use. This dish has been adapted from a recipe on www.alprosoy.co.uk.

SERVES 1

For the Compote
- ¾ cup fresh or frozen raspberries (thawed)
- ¼ cup pomegranate juice
- honey to taste

For the Oatmeal
- ½ cup rolled oats
- 1 cup soy milk
- honey to taste

To make the compote, place the raspberries and the pomegranate juice in a saucepan. Bring to a boil and simmer for 5 minutes or until the liquid has reduced. Remove from the heat and stir in honey to taste.

To make the oatmeal, place the oats and milk in a medium-sized heatproof bowl and stir. Cook on full power in the microwave for 2 minutes, stir, and cook for another minute. Let stand for 1 minute, then stir in the honey to taste.

Loosen the consistency with more milk, if you like, and top with the compote.

Good source of polyphenols and soy. Source of vitamin E
PER PORTION: 363 CAL, 8.4G FAT, 1.5G SATURATED FAT

salmon kedgeree

This Indian-style breakfast makes a wonderful brunch to share with friends.

SERVES 4

- 14 ounces salmon fillets
- 1 tablespoon lemon juice
- 2 tablespoons and ½ teaspoon olive oil
- salt and pepper
- 3 eggs
- 1½ cups basmati rice
- ½ red chile or more to taste
- ½ teaspoon turmeric
- ½ teaspoon garam masala
- ¼ cup fresh parsley, chopped
- yogurt or soy yogurt, for serving (optional)

Preheat the oven to 300°F.

Wash the salmon fillets and place on a sheet of aluminum foil. Sprinkle with the lemon juice, ½ teaspoon olive oil, and salt and pepper, and let it sit for a few minutes.

Wrap the fish in the foil and cook in the oven for 15–20 minutes or until cooked through, then break into large flakes. Meanwhile, boil the eggs in water for 10 minutes until hard-boiled. Drain, peel, and chop into ½-inch pieces. Boil the rice for 10 minutes and drain.

Heat 2 tablespoons of olive oil in a pan and lightly stir-fry the chile for 30 seconds. Add the turmeric and heat, stirring, for 1–2 minutes. Remove the pan from the heat, add the rice, and stir into the turmeric until the rice is a soft yellow color.

Stir in the salmon, eggs, garam masala, and most of the parsley. Serve with yogurt and sprinkled with the remaining parsley.

Good source of oily fish. Source of selenium
PER PORTION: 579 CAL, 24.7G FAT, 4.6G SATURATED FAT

bagels with oven-roasted tomatoes and arugula

Oven-roasting cherry tomatoes gives them a wonderful, concentrated flavor. You can do this the day before if you prefer, ready to serve for breakfast the next day. This dish has been selected from www.eggrecipes.co.uk.

SERVES 4

- 1 pound cherry tomatoes, cut in half
- 1 tablespoon olive oil
- 4 large eggs
- 4 bagels, split
- large handful of wild arugula leaves
- salt and freshly ground black pepper

Preheat the oven to 300°F.

Place the tomatoes, cut side up, on a baking tray, drizzle the oil over them, and season with salt and pepper. Bake for 35–40 minutes or until the tomatoes have shriveled and dried out a little.

Fill a large frying pan with salted water and bring to a boil. Carefully crack the eggs into the simmering water, then reduce the heat and cook for 3–5 minutes, depending upon how you like your eggs poached. Lift the eggs from the water with a slotted spoon and drain on paper towels.

Meanwhile, toast the bagels. To serve, place each bagel on a plate. Top with the tomatoes, arugula, and a poached egg.

Season to taste with salt and pepper, and serve immediately.

Source of cruciferous vegetables and lycopene
PER PORTION: 317 CAL, 10.6G FAT, 2.4G SATURATED FAT

dried shiitake mushroom and tomato omelet

This omelet makes a satisfying cooked breakfast and is great served with wholewheat toast and British Heinz baked beans.

SERVES 1

- 10g sun-dried shiitake mushrooms, soaked in hot water for a half hour
- 2 teaspoons olive oil spread
- 1½ tablespoons sun-dried tomatoes in oil, drained and chopped
- 2 eggs
- 1 tablespoon water
- salt and pepper

Preheat the broiler to hot.

Drain and slice the soaked mushrooms and remove any hard stalks. Melt the spread in a frying pan. Add the mushrooms and sauté until golden brown. Add the tomatoes and heat through.

Meanwhile, whisk together the eggs and water, and season with salt and pepper. Add the egg mixture to the mushrooms and tomatoes, and stir gently.

Draw the set mixture from the sides of the frying pan into the middle and let the liquid mixture run to the sides. When the omelet has set, place the frying pan under the hot broiler to brown the top.

Source of lycopene, vitamin D, vitamin E, and selenium
PER PORTION: 290 CAL, 22.1G FAT, 5.6G SATURATED FAT

apricot and brazil nut breakfast bars

These delicious breakfast bars are easy to make and can be kept in the fridge for days to grab as a quick breakfast or healthy snack. The Brazil nuts provide plenty of selenium, and as there is no added fat, they are healthier than most cereal bars.

MAKES 14

- 1 cup dried apricots
- 1¼ cups Brazil nuts
- ⅓ cup dark chocolate chips
- ½ cup rolled oats
- ½ cup muesli
- 1 cup puffed rice cereal
- 3 tablespoons honey
- ⅓ cup orange juice

Preheat the oven to 350°F.

Chop the dried apricots and Brazil nuts into small pieces of irregular size. Place all the dry ingredients in a mixing bowl and mix well. Next, stir in the honey and orange juice until evenly combined.

Line a jelly-roll pan (12 x 7-inch) with parchment paper and spoon in the mixture. Smooth down with the back of a spoon so the mixture is tightly packed and of even thickness.

Place in the oven for 20 minutes; check after 15 minutes to ensure it does not burn. Remove from the oven and let cool for an hour or two, then chill in the fridge overnight.

Cut into 14 bars and store in the fridge.

Good source of selenium
PER BAR: 162 CAL, 9.0G FAT, 2.4G SATURATED FAT

cranberry and brazil nut breakfast bars

These are an equally tasty variation of the Apricot and Brazil Nut Breakfast Bars.

MAKES 14

- 1 cup dried cranberries
- 1¼ cups Brazil nuts
- ½ cup rolled oats
- ½ cup muesli
- 1 cup puffed rice cereal
- 3 tablespoons honey
- ⅓ cup pomegranate or apple juice

Preheat the oven to 350°F.

Chop the cranberries and Brazil nuts into small pieces of irregular size. Place all the dry ingredients in a mixing bowl and mix well. Next, stir in the honey and fruit juice until evenly combined.

Line a jelly-roll pan (12 x 7-inch) with parchment paper and spoon in the mixture. Smooth down with the back of a spoon so the mixture is tightly packed and of even thickness.

Place in the oven for 20 minutes; check after 15 minutes to ensure it does not burn. Remove from the oven and let cool for an hour or two, then chill in the fridge overnight.

Cut into 14 bars and store in the fridge.

Good source of selenium
PER BAR: 158 CAL, 8.0G FAT, 1.8G SATURATED FAT

soups,
appetizers,
and dips

caribbean pepperpot

Garnished with peppers, this soup is vibrant, fragrant, and colorful. It is also packed with beneficial vegetables. This recipe has been selected from *The New Cranks Recipe Book* by Nadine Abensur.

SERVES 4

- ⅓ cup sunflower oil
- 1¼ cups onions, chopped
- 3 garlic cloves, finely chopped
- 2 cups cubed potatoes
- ½ bouillon cube, dissolved in 1 cup hot water
- 1⅔ cups chopped green cabbage
- 1 x 14½-oz. can diced tomatoes
- 1 heaping tablespoon paprika
- 1 heaping teaspoon ground coriander
- dash of Tabasco
- ½ teaspoon ground chile powder
- 1 fresh chile, finely chopped
- 1 x 14½-oz. can coconut milk
- pinch of soft brown sugar (optional)

For the Peppers
- 1 tablespoon sunflower oil
- 1 red pepper, cubed
- 1 yellow pepper, cubed
- dash of Tabasco
- 1–2 tablespoons tamari (wheat-free soy sauce)

In a large pot, heat the oil and sauté the onions and garlic until transparent.

Add the cubed potatoes until they, too, are transparent. Add ¼ cup of the hot bouillon, stir, and cook for 1 minute or so. Then add the chopped cabbage and sauté for 2–3 minutes. Drain the canned tomatoes, reserving the juice. Add the tomatoes to the soup along with the paprika, ground coriander, Tabasco, and chile powder. Stir well and add the remaining hot bouillon, the reserved tomato juice, and fresh chile. Simmer gently for 7–8 minutes and add the coconut milk.

Check the sweetness of the soup and, if necessary, add a pinch of soft brown sugar. For the peppers, heat the oil in a frying pan and sauté the peppers for just a minute, until they begin to blacken in places. Add a drop or two of Tabasco and tamari to taste, and set aside.

To serve, mix half the peppers into the soup and reserve the rest to use as garnish on each serving, or in the soup tureen.

Good source of Allium vegetables. Source of cruciferous vegetables, lycopene, and vitamin E
PER PORTION: 332 CAL, 20.9G FAT, 3.1G SATURATED FAT

armenian soup

This soup has a wonderful and unusual flavor and goes well with the Peanut and Flaxseed Bread (page 76). This recipe has been kindly provided by Jo Dilley.

SERVES 4

- ⅓ cup red lentils, washed
- ⅓ cup ready-to-eat dried apricots
- 1 medium potato, chopped
- 5 cups vegetable broth
- juice of half a lemon
- 1 teaspoon ground cumin
- salt and pepper
- 3 tablespoons fresh parsley plus extra sprigs, for serving
- ¼ cup yogurt or soy yogurt (optional), for serving

Put all the ingredients except the yogurt and the extra sprigs of parsley into a large pot and bring to a boil. Reduce the heat, cover, and simmer for 30 minutes.

Let the soup cool, then blend in a food processor or blender until smooth. Reheat and adjust the seasoning before serving.

Garnish each bowl with a swirl of yogurt and a sprig of parsley.

Source of legumes
PER PORTION: 137 CAL, 2.7G FAT, 0.2G SATURATED FAT

fava bean soup

Serve this delicious summer soup with crusty homemade bread. You can substitute the fava beans with peas if you prefer. This recipe has been kindly provided by Dr. John Rayman.

SERVES 4–6

- 2 tablespoons olive oil
- 1 bunch of scallions, chopped
- 18 ounces frozen or fresh fava beans
- ¼ cup parsley, chopped
- 1¾ cups soy milk
- salt and pepper
- pinch of nutmeg
- soy cream, for serving (optional)

If the fava beans are large, with tough outer skins, blanch them for 1 minute and drain. Then pop them out of their skins and simply continue with the recipe as follows.

Heat the oil in a large saucepan and gently cook the scallions until they are soft. Add the beans and parsley and just enough water to cover the beans. Bring to a boil, cover, and simmer for 5–10 minutes or until the beans are cooked.

Let the soup cool and then blend to a puree in a food processor or blender. In a clean pan, stir the puree into the milk and heat gently without boiling. Add salt, pepper, and nutmeg, to taste. Serve with a swirl of soy cream if you like.

Good source of legumes. Source of **Allium** *vegetables and soy*
PER PORTION: 171 CAL, 10G FAT, 1.5G SATURATED FAT

chilled tomato bisque

This recipe has been kindly provided by Antony Worrall Thompson. It is based on gazpacho but is smooth instead of chunky. It is wonderfully refreshing on a hot summer's day.

SERVES 4

- 1 slice wholewheat bread, crusts removed and broken into large crumbs
- 1 tablespoon sherry vinegar
- 1 garlic clove, peeled and finely chopped
- 1 teaspoon sugar
- ½ red chile, seeded and finely chopped
- 2 tablespoons extra virgin olive oil
- 1 x 14½-oz. can tomatoes
- scant cup tomato juice
- 2 scallions, finely sliced
- ½ red pepper, roasted or broiled, peeled, seeded, and cubed
- ½ large cucumber, peeled, seeded, and roughly chopped
- 2 teaspoons pesto
- salt and freshly ground black pepper

Place the bread in a food processor or blender. With the machine running add the vinegar, garlic, sugar, and chile, and blend until smooth. Add the extra virgin olive oil until the bread will absorb no more, then, a little at a time, add the tomatoes, tomato juice, scallions, red pepper, cucumber, and pesto.

Continue to blend to form a smooth emulsion. Season to taste with salt and black pepper, and transfer to a large bowl. Ladle into chilled soup bowls and serve immediately.

Good source of lycopene. Source of **Allium** *vegetables*
PER PORTION: 138 CAL, 9.1G FAT, 1.5G SATURATED FAT

roasted tomato and sweet potato soup

Roasting the tomatoes and sweet potato enhances their beautiful flavors. Serve this delicious soup with Brazil Nut, Tomato, and Onion Bread (page 74).

SERVES 4

- 1 pound sweet potatoes, peeled and sliced
- 2½ pounds tomatoes, cut in half
- 2 tablespoons olive oil
- 1 large onion, chopped into wedges
- 2 garlic cloves, sliced
- salt and pepper
- 1 small bunch basil leaves, torn, plus extra for garnishing
- 1 tablespoon tomato paste

Preheat the oven to 400°F.

Parboil the potatoes in a saucepan for 5 minutes, then drain, and let cool. Combine all the ingredients except for the tomato paste and oil, and place on a roasting tray. Drizzle with the oil.

Roast in the oven for 30 minutes, turning the vegetables halfway through. Once removed from the oven, pick any burnt skins off the tomatoes which will come away easily.

Blend all the ingredients along with 2½ cups water and the tomato paste in a blender or food processor. Reheat to serve, and garnish with a few basil leaves.

Good source of Allium *vegetables and lycopene. Source of vitamin E*
PER PORTION: 236 CAL, 7.9G FAT, 1.4G SATURATED FAT

winter vegetable soup

For this heart-warming soup, why not try varying the vegetables? You could use parsnips, cabbage, or whatever you like, but keep the leeks and onion in it to get a good source of *Allium* vegetables.

SERVES 6

- 2 tablespoons olive oil spread
- 2 leeks, sliced
- 2 carrots, peeled and chopped
- 1 potato, peeled and chopped
- 1 rutabaga, peeled and chopped
- 1 onion, chopped
- 2 tablespoons fresh herbs, chopped
- 6 cups vegetable or chicken broth
- salt and pepper

Melt the olive oil spread in a large pot and add all the ingredients except the stock. Cover and heat gently for 20 minutes, stirring occasionally. If the vegetables begin to stick, add a few tablespoons of water, then add the broth, cover, and simmer for another 10 minutes or until the vegetables are tender.

Let cool, then place in a food processor or blender and blend until smooth. Season with salt and pepper to taste. You may want to set aside a few pieces of the chopped, cooked vegetables for garnishing. Reheat to serve.

Good source of Allium *vegetables. Source of cruciferous vegetables*
PER PORTION: 91 CAL, 4.2G FAT, 0.7G SATURATED FAT

watercress soup

The watercress gives this soup a lovely peppery taste which works well with the dairy-free cream. This dish has been adapted from a recipe on www.alprosoy.co.uk.

SERVES 4

- 1 medium onion, finely chopped
- 1 tablespoon olive oil
- ½ pound new potatoes, peeled and chopped
- 2 large bunches of watercress
- 1¾ cups vegetable broth
- 1 cup dairy-free alternative to light cream

In a large saucepan, cook the onion in the olive oil until soft. Add the peeled and chopped potatoes and cook for 2 minutes. Add the watercress, then pour in the boiling stock.

Bring back to a boil and then simmer for 15–20 minutes, until the potatoes are cooked. Blend the soup while adding the cream, reserving 1 tablespoon for serving. Adjust seasoning and serve with a swirl of cream to finish it.

Source of Allium *and cruciferous vegetables and soy*
PER PORTION: 226 CAL, 6.4G FAT, 2.2G SATURATED FAT

tiger shrimp and shiitake mushroom broth

This recipe was created by TV chef Alex Mackay. Here's what he has to say about it:

"This very pretty soup is both fresh and refreshing, with a little bite from the ginger and a fresh burst of mint at the end. Shrimp are delightful with soy, somehow standing up to the strength of the sauce and soothing it at the same time. The peppers and honey help too, giving the soup a gentle suggestion of sweetness."

SERVES 4

- 12 whole tiger shrimp, head and shell on
- 2 lemon grass sticks, finely chopped
- 3 tablespoons grated ginger (no need to peel it)
- 2 tablespoons tomato paste
- 2 tablespoons soy sauce
- 2 tablespoons honey
- 6 cups chicken broth (or vegetable bouillon)
- 2 small red peppers, cut in half, seeded, and chopped into small chunks
- 4 garlic cloves, peeled and chopped
- 1 bunch of scallions, roots trimmed, and sliced on an angle
- 12 dried shiitake mushrooms, soaked, and thickly sliced
- 2 heads of bok choy, cut into quarters
- 6–7 ounces medium egg noodles (2 of the squares from a package)
- 5 sprigs of mint leaves, picked from their stalks and sliced

Remove the shells and heads from the shrimp and put them into a large pot. Remove the veins from the shrimp tails and set aside. To the pot, add the lemon grass, ginger, tomato paste, soy sauce, honey, and stock. Bring to a boil and simmer rapidly for 15 minutes.

Strain the stock into a clean pot. Add the peppers and garlic. Bring to a boil, lower the heat, and simmer for 5 minutes. Bring a large pot of water to a boil for the noodles. Add the shrimp, scallions, mushrooms, and bok choy to the stock and poach gently for 5–6 minutes, making sure the liquid never boils. In the other pot, boil the noodles for 3–4 minutes and strain into a colander. Scoop into soup bowls and top with the shrimp, vegetables, and mint. Boil the broth and ladle it over the top.

Good source of Allium *and cruciferous vegetables. Source of lycopene and vitamins E and D*
PER PORTION: 364 CAL, 6.1G FAT, 1.5G SATURATED FAT

pea and mint soup

This pretty, bright green soup should be blended well for a smooth and creamy texture. It makes a satisfying lunch served with crusty bread. This recipe has been kindly provided by Dr. John Rayman.

SERVES 4

- 1½ cups chopped onion
- 1 cup chopped potatoes
- 1 tablespoon olive oil
- 5 cups vegetable (or chicken) stock
- 1 pound frozen peas, defrosted
- 1 bunch of mint, chopped
- 1¼ cups soy milk
- salt and pepper
- a little soy cream and a few mint leaves, for garnishing

Cook the onion and potato in the olive oil for 5 minutes until soft (but not browned). Add the stock, bring to a boil, and simmer for 20 minutes or until the potato is soft. Add the peas, return to a boil, and simmer for 2 minutes.

Add the mint and then immediately puree in a blender until the soup is smooth. Add the soy milk. Season with salt and pepper and then reheat gently before serving.

Garnish with a swirl of soy cream and a few mint leaves.

Good source of legumes. Source of Allium **vegetables and soy**
PER PORTION: 184 CAL, 6.8G FAT, 0.9G SATURATED FAT

roasted cauliflower and carrot soup

Roasting the vegetables brings out the sweet flavors in this thick and creamy soup.

SERVES 6

- ½ pound carrots, peeled and chopped
- 2 tablespoons olive oil
- salt and pepper
- 1¼ pounds cauliflower, chopped into florets
- 3 garlic cloves, chopped
- 1 medium onion, chopped
- 5 cups vegetable or chicken stock
- 1 teaspoon grated nutmeg
- paprika, for serving

Preheat the oven to 350°F.

Place the carrots on a roasting tray, toss in half a tablespoon of the oil, and sprinkle with salt and pepper. Roast for 10 minutes. Remove from the oven, add the cauliflower florets and another half tablespoon of oil to the tray. Return to the oven for another 20 minutes.

Meanwhile heat the remaining tablespoon of oil in a large pot over medium heat and cook the garlic and onions for 5 minutes. Pour in the stock and simmer for 5 minutes. Finally, add the roasted vegetables and nutmeg, and simmer for 5 minutes more.

Remove from the heat and let cool, then blend until smooth. Reheat and sprinkle with paprika when ready to serve.

Good source of cruciferous vegetables. Source of Allium **vegetables**
PER PORTION: 103 CAL, 6.1G FAT, 1.0G SATURATED FAT

french onion soup

This hearty soup is marvelous on a cold and wet autumn evening. This recipe has been kindly provided by Dr. John Rayman.

SERVES 4

- 2¼ pounds onions, sliced
- 1 tablespoon olive oil
- 4 cups beef stock
- salt and pepper

For the Croutons
- 2 garlic cloves, crushed
- 1 tablespoon olive oil
- 4 slices stale bread, crusts removed, cut into ½-inch cubes
- Gruyère cheese, grated, for serving (optional)

Preheat the oven to 400°F.

Cook the onions gently in the olive oil in a large pot until they are golden brown. Add the stock and season with salt and pepper. Bring to a boil and simmer, covered, for about 45 minutes.

To make the croutons, cook the garlic and bread in the olive oil in a frying pan for a couple of minutes.

Turn the contents of the frying pan onto a cookie sheet and place in the oven for about 10 minutes or until the croutons are browned. Serve the soup topped with the croutons and some grated Gruyère, if you like.

Good source of Allium vegetables
PER PORTION: 122 CAL, 4.7G FAT, 0.5G SATURATED FAT

brazil nut, tomato, and onion bread

This bread has a lovely texture and is great with soup. Try sprinkling other seeds on the top of the loaves such as cumin, caraway, or fennel. This bread also freezes very well. The recipe has been kindly provided by Dr. John Rayman.

MAKES 10 SLICES PER LOAF

- 3 medium onions, chopped
- 2 tablespoons olive oil
- ⅔ cup Brazil nuts, chopped
- 1¾ ounces sun-dried tomatoes, chopped
- 2¼ cups wholegrain rye flour
- 3¼ cups white bread flour
- 2 teaspoons salt
- 1 envelope dry yeast
- 2 cups water
- milk for glazing
- 4 teaspoons poppy seeds

Preheat the oven to 425°F.

Cook the onions gently in the olive oil in a frying pan until they are soft and light brown. Place the nuts, tomatoes, flours, salt, and yeast in the bowl of a food processor (using a dough hook if you have one) and add the entire contents of the frying pan. Mix for a few seconds to blend in the oil.

Boil ⅔ cup of the water and mix with the remaining cold water and add to the mixture. Knead by hand or blend in the food processor using the dough hook, until you have a smooth dough. You may need to add a little more water at this stage; don't worry if the dough becomes a little sloppy. Put the dough into a large bowl, cover with plastic wrap, and leave in a warm place until the volume of the dough has doubled.

Grease two 8 x 4 x 2-inch loaf pans. Knead the dough briskly for a few minutes. Divide the dough into two equal parts and place each half in a loaf pan. Cover the pans with plastic wrap and leave until the volume of the dough has doubled again. Brush the loaves with milk and sprinkle the poppy seeds on top. Put the loaves into the hot oven and bake for 30 minutes. Remove the loaves from their pans and bake for another 10 minutes or until a skewer stuck into the bread comes out clean. Let cool on a wire rack.

Good source of selenium. Source of Allium vegetables and lycopene
PER SLICE: 186 CAL, 6.3G FAT, 1.1G SATURATED FAT

peanut and flaxseed bread

Although this recipe only meets our criteria as a source of vitamin E, it contains legumes (peanuts) and phytoestrogens as lignans (flaxseeds and rye). To give the bread a coarser texture, you can replace some of the white flour with wholegrain or wholewheat flour, or add a tablespoon of seeds to the flour mixture. This bread freezes very well.

MAKES 10 SLICES PER LOAF

- 1 cup salted peanuts, chopped coarsely
- ⅔ cup flaxseeds, briefly ground in a grinder
- 1 cup sunflower seeds
- 1½ cups wholegrain rye flour
- 4 cups white bread flour
- 1 tablespoon olive oil
- 2 teaspoons salt
- 1 envelope dry yeast
- 2 cups water
- milk for glazing
- 4 teaspoons caraway seeds
- sunflower, sesame, pumpkin, or hemp seeds (optional)

Preheat the oven to 425°F.

Blend the peanuts briefly in a food processor to give a coarse ground mixture. Grind the flaxseeds in a coffee grinder for 10–15 seconds. Place the peanuts, flaxseeds, sunflower seeds, flours, olive oil, salt, and yeast in the bowl of a food processor (using a dough hook if you have one). Mix to blend in the oil. Boil ⅔ cup of the water and mix with the remaining cold water and add to the mixture. Knead or blend in the food processor until you have a smooth dough. You may need to add a little more water; don't worry if the dough becomes a little sloppy.

Put the dough in a large bowl, cover with plastic wrap, and leave in a warm place until the volume of the dough has doubled. Grease two 8 x 4 x 2-inch loaf pans. With floured hands, knead the dough briskly for a few minutes, then divide into two equal parts and place each half in a loaf pan. Cover the pans with plastic wrap and leave until the dough volume has doubled again. Brush the loaves with milk and sprinkle the caraway seeds on top. Put the loaves into the oven and bake for 30 minutes. Remove the loaves from the pans and bake for 10 minutes more until a skewer stuck into the bread comes out clean. Let cool on a wire rack.

Source of vitamin E
PER SLICE: 235 CAL, 9.9G FAT, 1.3G SATURATED FAT

fava bean and apple crostini

Crostini are great as an appetizer or as a lunch dish with salad. For an attractive appetizer plate serve these with the Sweet Tomato and Chile Crostini (opposite page).

SERVES 4–6

- 1 small baguette cut into 12 slices about ¾-inch thick
- 1 tablespoon olive oil

For the Fava bean and Apple Topping
- 7 ounces frozen fava beans
- 1 tablespoon crunchy peanut butter
- 1–2 tablespoons water
- 4 scallions, sliced
- 1 small red apple, chopped
- salt and pepper

Preheat the oven to 400°F.

Brush the bread slices on both sides with the olive oil and place on a baking tray. Place in the oven for about 10 minutes or until the bread is golden brown. Remove from the oven and let cool.

Cook the fava beans in boiling water for about 5 minutes. Drain and set aside until cool enough to handle. Remove the skins from the fava beans and discard. Place two thirds of the fava beans in a bowl and mash with a fork. Mix in the peanut butter and enough water to make a soft paste.

Stir in the remaining fava beans, scallions, and apple, and season to taste. Spread a generous amount of topping on each of the bread slices and serve.

Source of legumes
PER PORTION: 290 CAL, 10.9G FAT, 1.8G SATURATED FAT

sweet tomato and chile crostini

The sweet chile sauce works well with the tomatoes in this recipe. For an attractive appetizer plate, serve these with the Fava bean and Apple Crostini (opposite page).

SERVES 4–6

- 1 small baguette cut into 12 slices about ¾ inch thick
- 1 tablespoon olive oil

For the Tomato and Chile Topping
- 1 teaspoon olive oil
- 1 small red onion, finely chopped
- 2 garlic cloves, crushed
- 1½ ounces sun-dried tomatoes, finely chopped
- 2 fresh tomatoes, chopped
- 2 teaspoons sweet chile sauce, or more to taste
- salt and pepper

Preheat the oven to 400°F.

Brush the bread slices on both sides with the olive oil and place on a baking tray. Place in the oven for about 10 minutes or until the bread is golden brown. Remove from the oven and let cool.

Heat the oil for the topping in a small frying pan, add the onion and garlic, and cook until soft. Next add the sun-dried tomatoes and continue to cook for a couple of minutes more. Remove from the heat and let cool. Put the chopped tomatoes in a bowl and stir in the onion mixture. Add the sweet chile sauce, stir to combine, and season to taste. Heap a generous mound of topping onto each bread slice and serve.

Good source of lycopene. Source of Allium *vegetables and vitamin E*
PER PORTION: 270 CAL, 11.7G FAT, 1.8G SATURATED FAT

dr. john's liver terrine

This is a dish of Ashkenazi Jewish origin, traditionally served with Jewish unleavened bread known as matzos. It can be served with additional onions browned in olive oil and allowed to cool. You can decorate it with chopped hard-boiled eggs. Chicken livers can be substituted for some of the lamb liver, and the proportions of liver, egg, and onion can be adjusted to taste. This recipe has been kindly provided by Dr. John Rayman.

SERVES 10

- 1½ pounds lamb liver, sliced
- 2 cups chicken broth
- 5 medium eggs
- 1 tablespoon olive oil
- 2¼ cups onion, chopped
- salt and pepper

In a large pan gently poach the liver in the chicken stock until it is cooked. Remove from the heat and let cool in the pan. Hard boil the eggs by boiling them in water for 10 minutes. Drain and let cool, then remove the shells.

Heat the oil in a frying pan and cook the onions until golden brown, then remove from the heat and let cool in the pan. Either grind the eggs, liver, and onion together using a meat grinder, or else use a food processor in short pulses to produce a rough-textured terrine, not a smooth pâté.

Season to taste with salt and pepper and enough of the chicken stock to ensure that the terrine is moist.

Source of **Allium** *vegetables and selenium*
PER PORTION: 165 CAL, 8.8G FAT, 2.2G SATURATED FAT

POM salsa

This pomegranate salsa is excellent served with tortilla chips and will keep, covered, in the fridge for 2 to 3 days. The recipe has been selected from www.pomwonderful.com.

SERVES 4

- 2–3 large pomegranates
- 3½ tablespoons pomegranate juice
- 3–4 teaspoons jalapeño pepper, chopped
- ⅓ cup finely chopped yellow pepper
- 4 tablespoons cilantro, chopped
- 1 tablespoon granulated sugar
- 1 tablespoon rice vinegar

Score 2–3 fresh pomegranates and place in a bowl of water.

Break open the pomegranates under water to free the arils (red seed sacs). The arils will sink to the bottom of the bowl and the membrane will float to the top. Strain the arils and put them in a separate bowl. Leftover arils can be refrigerated or frozen to use another time. Put all the ingredients in a large bowl and thoroughly mix to combine.

Good source of polyphenols
PER PORTION: 71 CAL, 0.3G FAT, 0.0G SATURATED FAT

cooked tomato salsa

This salsa is good served warm or chilled and makes a great accompaniment to cooked meats and salad.

SERVES 4

- 1 tablespoon olive oil
- 1 bunch of scallions, sliced
- 2 garlic cloves, chopped
- 2 cups chopped tomatoes
- juice of half a lime
- 1 teaspoon sugar
- salt and pepper

Gently heat the olive oil in a frying pan. Add the onions and garlic, and lightly cook for about 5 minutes until the onions are soft and golden.

Add the tomatoes and cook for another 5 minutes. Add the lime juice and sugar and continue cooking for 1–2 minutes more.

Season to taste with salt and pepper and serve, or chill in the fridge for later.

Source of Allium **vegetables and lycopene**
PER PORTION: 60 CAL, 3.9G FAT, 0.6G SATURATED FAT

fava bean puree

This fresh fava bean recipe is taken from *Moro: The Cookbook* by Sam and Sam Clark. It was inspired by the classic, earthy Egyptian fava bean puree (made with dried fava beans). Serve as an appetizer with pita bread or as part of a mezze.

SERVES 4

- 2¼ pounds fresh fava beans, shelled (or 2 cups already shelled)
- 1 garlic clove, crushed to a paste with salt
- a squeeze of lemon
- 2 tablespoons olive oil
- 1 small bunch of fresh mint, roughly chopped
- sea salt or kosher salt and black pepper

Bring a saucepan of unsalted water to a boil and add the fresh shelled fava beans. Cook for about 5 minutes or until soft.

Drain, then transfer to a food processor or food mill, and puree until smooth. Transfer to a bowl, then add the garlic, lemon juice, olive oil, and mint, and season with salt and pepper. If the texture is a little thick, stir in some extra oil or water.

Source of Allium **vegetables and legumes**
PER PORTION: 141 CAL, 7.9G FAT, 1.1G SATURATED FAT

salads

chickpea salad

This salad can be served as part of a mixed salad plate or as an accompaniment to fish or poultry. This recipe has been kindly provided by Suzanne Burton.

SERVES 4–6

- 1⅓ cups bulgur, prepared according to package instructions
- 1¾ ounces dried apricots, finely chopped
- 1 red onion, finely chopped
- 1 x 15-oz. can chickpeas, drained and rinsed
- 1¾ ounces sun-dried tomatoes in oil, drained and chopped
- 1 bunch of scallions, sliced
- 1 large handful of cilantro, chopped
- 1 cup pitted black olives
- 4 tablespoons sunflower seeds
- salt and pepper

For the Dressing
- juice of 1 lemon
- 2 tablespoons olive oil
- 2 garlic cloves, crushed

Put the prepared bulgur in a large bowl. Stir in the remaining salad ingredients, except the seasoning. Combine the dressing ingredients and stir into the salad. Season to taste.

Good source of legumes and lycopene. Source of Allium vegetables, vitamin E, and selenium
PER PORTION: 525 CAL, 20.5G FAT, 2.3G SATURATED FAT

greek salad

This is a pretty-looking salad which couldn't be easier to make. It can be served as a light, summery side dish and makes a welcome addition to a buffet.

SERVES 6

- 4 tomatoes
- 1 red onion
- 1 cucumber
- 5 ounces feta cheese
- 1 x 15-oz. can chickpeas, drained
- 1 tablespoon mint sauce or a handful of fresh mint, chopped

Chop the tomatoes, onion, cucumber, and feta cheese into cubes of uniform size, about the size of a chickpea. Place all the ingredients in a large bowl and mix well.

Source of Allium vegetables, legumes, and lycopene
PER PORTION: 132 CAL, 6.5G FAT, 3.6G SATURATED FAT

salmon vermicelli salad

This dish was kindly provided by Dr. Sophie Chen, Research Director of the Ovarian and Prostate Cancer Research Trust Laboratory. It is really tasty and packed with beneficial ingredients.

SERVES 2

- 1¾ ounces dry vermicelli, rice or mung bean noodles
- ²/₃ cup grated carrot
- 6 ounces mung bean sprouts
- 3 ounces watercress or arugula
- 2 salmon fillets, broiled or baked
- 1 cup shredded crispy seaweed

For the Sauce
- 2 tablespoons olive oil
- 2 tablespoons balsamic vinegar
- 2 tablespoons soy sauce
- 3–4 garlic cloves, chopped
- ½ teaspoon sesame oil (optional)
- 1 tablespoon lemon juice (optional)

Prepare the vermicelli according to the package instructions. Cut into shorter pieces, and place in a large bowl. Add the carrot and mung bean sprouts.

Combine the sauce ingredients in another bowl and mix well. Add two thirds of the sauce to the vermicelli mixture and put aside. Layer the watercress or arugula on a plate, followed by a layer of the vermicelli mixture.

Place the salmon on top of the vermicelli salad and pour the remaining sauce over it. Finally, sprinkle the crispy seaweed on top.

Good source of Allium vegetables, oily fish, legumes, and vitamin D. Source of cruciferous vegetables, selenium, and vitamin E
PER PORTION: 494 CAL, 27.2G FAT, 4.7G SATURATED FAT

mediterranean pasta salad

This colorful dish is a real taste of the Mediterranean and goes down well as part of a buffet. As well as tasting great, the sun-dried tomatoes will give you a big dose of lycopene!

SERVES 10–20

- 18 ounces pasta bows
- ¼ cup olive oil
- 1 tablespoon white wine vinegar
- 1 tablespoon tomato paste
- 1 tablespoon red pesto
- 1 small jar sun-dried tomatoes in olive oil, drained and chopped
- handful of pitted black olives, cut in half
- a few basil leaves, shredded

Boil the pasta according to the package instructions and drain.

Mix together the oil, white wine vinegar, tomato paste, and red pesto, and stir into the pasta. Simply combine with the remaining ingredients and serve at room temperature.

Good source of lycopene
PER PORTION: 264 CAL, 9.1G FAT, 1.3G SATURATED FAT

asian salad

This is a delightful, crunchy salad full of beneficial foods. The tofu provides a good source of soy, but if you prefer you could use cooked chicken breast instead.

SERVES 4

- a few handfuls of salad greens
- 3 large tomatoes
- 1 cucumber, peeled and cut into wedges
- 1 head broccoli, chopped into very small florets
- ½ red pepper, cut into thin strips
- 2 medium onions, cut into fine rings
- 3 hard-boiled eggs, chopped into wedges
- half a bunch cilantro
- 12 ounces tofu, cubed

For the Dressing
- ⅔ cup unsalted, roasted peanuts
- ½ cup lemon juice
- 3 tablespoons white wine vinegar
- 4 garlic cloves
- 3 tablespoons chopped cilantro and stalks
- 3 tablespoons sugar
- 1 teaspoon salt
- 1 tablespoon water
- 1 whole chile
- 1 tablespoon fish sauce

For the dressing, blend all the ingredients together in a blender or food processor. Pour into a large bowl.

Place the salad greens on four plates and toss all of the other salad ingredients into the dressing. Lay the salad on the bed of greens and serve.

Good source of **Allium** *and cruciferous vegetables and soy. Source of lycopene, legumes, and vitamin E*
PER PORTION: 383 CAL, 19.2G FAT, 3.8G SATURATED FAT

mixed bean salad

With a variety of different beans, this salad, which can be prepared in five minutes, is a tasty way to top up on legumes.

SERVES 6

- 6 ounces frozen baby fava beans
- 4 ounces young green beans
- 1 x 14-oz. can mixed beans, drained
- ¾ cup canned corn, drained
- 1 tablespoon olive oil
- 2 teaspoons white wine vinegar
- 1 tablespoon wholegrain mustard

Boil the fava beans and green beans in a pan of water for 5 minutes or until cooked. Drain and let cool.

Mix all the ingredients in a bowl and serve.

Good source of legumes
PER PORTION: 100 CAL, 3.1G FAT, 0.4G SATURATED FAT

POM vinaigrette

Since only a small quantity of vinaigrette is used to dress a salad, this recipe does not meet any of our "source of" or "good source of" criteria. However, it is an excellent way to serve up some extra pomegranate juice and *Allium* vegetables. This vinaigrette can be made up to two days before serving and kept in the fridge. This recipe has been selected from www.pomwonderful.com.

MAKES ABOUT 1 CUP

- ⅓ cup pomegranate juice
- 2 ounces pomegranate arils (optional)
- ¼ cup olive oil
- ⅓ cup red or white wine vinegar
- 2 tablespoons grated red onion
- ½ teaspoon sugar, or to taste
- ½ teaspoon salt
- ⅛ teaspoon freshly ground pepper

In a screw-top jar or a plastic container with a tight-fitting lid, combine all of the dressing ingredients. Cover and shake well. Set aside or refrigerate before serving.

PER PORTION (2 TABLESPOONS): 76 CAL, 7.5G FAT, 1.1G SATURATED FAT

tiger shrimp salad with mango and avocado

Look for the largest, freshest tiger shrimp at the fish market—they need little cooking, and taste divine. This dish has been selected from *Gordon Ramsay Makes It Easy* by Gordon Ramsay.

SERVES 2

- 12 raw tiger shrimp, peeled, heads removed
- 1 large ripe mango, peeled and pit removed
- 1 large ripe avocado, peeled
- juice of half a lemon
- 1 tablespoon olive oil
- ½-inch piece fresh ginger root, peeled
- 1 garlic clove, peeled
- juice of 1 lime
- sea salt or kosher salt, and pepper
- 1 tablespoon flat-leaf parsley, chopped

De-vein the shrimp if necessary. Puree half the mango flesh in a blender or food processor and set aside. Cube the rest of the mango.

Cut the avocado in half, remove the pit, and slice the flesh. Arrange the slices around the outside of a small platter and drizzle the lemon juice over them. Heat the oil in a large frying pan, add the ginger and garlic, and cook for 30 seconds.

Add the shrimp and stir-fry for 2–3 minutes, until they turn pink —don't overcook. Drizzle with the lime juice and remove from the heat. Discard the ginger and garlic.

Add the cubed mango to the shrimp and toss together. Season with salt and pepper to taste. Pile the shrimp and mango in the middle of the platter and scatter the parsley over it. Drizzle the mango puree around the edge of the plate and serve.

Source of selenium and vitamin E
PER PORTION: 365 CAL, 26.3G FAT, 5.1G SATURATED FAT

salad niçoise

This French-style salad is delicious served with a crusty French baguette.

SERVES 4

- 2 eggs
- ¾ pound potatoes
- 4 ounces young green beans
- 11 ounces tuna steaks
- 1 teaspoon olive oil
- salt and pepper
- 3½ ounces arugula
- 4 tomatoes, cut into quarters
- 1 small onion, chopped or thinly sliced
- 1 x 2-oz. tin anchovy fillets in oil, drained
- handful of black olives

For the Dressing
- half a small bunch of fresh basil
- 1 garlic clove
- 2 tablespoons fresh lemon juice
- ¼ cup olive oil
- salt and pepper

Preheat the broiler to hot.

Boil the eggs in water for 10 minutes until hard-boiled. Drain and let cool. Peel and cut into sixths. In another pan, boil the potatoes for 20 minutes or until tender, adding the green beans for the last 5 minutes. Drain the potatoes and beans and run under cold water.

Chop the potatoes into bite-size pieces. Brush the tuna with 1 teaspoon of olive oil and rub with salt and pepper. Broil for about 2 minutes on each side. Let stand for a few minutes, then cut into cubes. To make the dressing, lower the basil leaves in a strainer into one of the pans of boiling water for a few seconds until wilted, then run under a cold tap. Blend the dressing ingredients together using a blender or food processor.

In a serving bowl, toss together the potatoes, beans, arugula, tomatoes, onion, and most of the dressing. Lay the egg and tuna on top, followed by the anchovies, then sprinkle with the olives and drizzle with the remaining dressing.

Good source of selenium. Source of **Allium** *and cruciferous vegetables, legumes, lycopene, oily fish, and vitamin E*
PER PORTION: 378 CAL, 22.7G FAT, 4.3G SATURATED FAT

cauliflower and broccoli salad

This salad can be served with couscous, warm pasta bows, or as part of a combined salad plate. Olives can be added, too—just stir them in at the end. This dish has been selected from *The New Cranks Recipe Book* by Nadine Abensur.

SERVES 6

- 1 large cauliflower, separated into florets
- 18 ounces broccoli, separated into florets
- 2 red peppers, charbroiled, peeled and thinly sliced

For the Dressing
- 3½ tablespoons extra-virgin olive oil
- 1 heaping tablespoon grain mustard
- ½ ounce fresh tarragon, picked off the stalks
- 4 garlic cloves, finely crushed
- dash of Tabasco
- dash of balsamic vinegar
- salt and freshly ground black pepper

Plunge the cauliflower and broccoli florets into a large pot of salted boiling water and blanch for 1 minute, until tender but still firm. Meanwhile combine the dressing ingredients.

Combine all the salad ingredients in a bowl and pour the dressing over them while the cauliflower and broccoli are still hot. Toss the salad, taste, and add more grain mustard if necessary.

Good source of cruciferous vegetables. Source of **Allium** *vegetables*
PER PORTION: 222 CAL, 18.8G FAT, 2.8G SATURATED FAT

main dishes

tuna stir-fry

This is a quick and easy meal to make. Try experimenting with different fish, e.g., salmon, and a variety of different beneficial vegetables. This dish has been adapted from a recipe by Jamie Oliver on www.sainsburys.co.uk.

SERVES 4

- 14 ounces fresh tuna steaks
- 3 tablespoons soy sauce
- 2-inch piece fresh ginger, peeled and grated
- small bunch of cilantro, finely chopped, keep some for garnish
- 2 fresh chiles, seeded and finely chopped
- 3½ ounces dried egg noodles
- 1 teaspoon sesame oil
- 1 tablespoon canola oil, plus a little extra to cook the tuna
- 4 scallions, finely sliced
- 1 garlic clove, peeled and finely sliced
- 1 carrot, peeled and shaved into strips with a peeler
- handful of sugar snap peas, sliced lengthways
- 1 red pepper, cut into strips
- ½ Chinese cabbage, thinly sliced
- large handful of fresh bean sprouts

Place the tuna in a bowl with the soy sauce, ginger, cilantro, and one of the red chiles, cover, and refrigerate for at least 20 minutes. Cook the noodles according to the package instructions, rinse with cold water, drain well, and toss in the sesame oil.

Remove the tuna to paper towels and reserve the marinade. Rub the tuna lightly with a little canola oil. Heat the grill pan and place the tuna in when hot. Cook on each side for 1–2 minutes, transfer to a plate, and keep warm.

Heat the canola oil in a wok. Add the scallions and garlic, and cook for a few seconds. Add the carrot, sugar snap peas, red peppers, cabbage, and bean sprouts. Stir-fry until slightly softened. Add the noodles and warm through. Add the leftover marinade and cook for a few seconds. Sprinkle with cilantro for serving.

Good source of oily fish and selenium. Source of **Allium** *vegetables, cruciferous vegetables, legumes, and vitamin D*
PER PORTION: 332 CAL, 11.2G FAT, 2.3G SATURATED FAT

tuna fish cakes

These fish cakes are very simple and taste wonderful whether you use salmon or tuna. They taste great on a hamburger bun with tomato ketchup and a salad.

SERVES 6

- 1¼ pounds potatoes, peeled and chopped
- 2 tablespoons olive oil
- 1 medium onion, grated
- 1 chile, finely chopped (or to taste)
- 1 teaspoon dried thyme
- 2 slices of bacon, finely chopped
- 1¼ pounds fresh tuna (or salmon)
- 1 egg, beaten
- salt and pepper
- flour for dusting

Boil the potatoes in a pan of water for 20 minutes or until tender. Drain and mash the potatoes. Heat 1 tablespoon of the oil in a frying pan and gently cook the onion, chile, thyme, and bacon for about 10 minutes or until the onions are soft. Set aside and let cool.

Coarsely chop the fish flesh with a knife or in a food processor. Mix all the ingredients together. Dust your hands with a little flour to avoid the mixture sticking to your hands and form into cakes. The mixture can either be made into 12 patties or into fish balls to serve as an appetizer.

Over a low heat, lightly fry the fish cakes on each side in the remaining tablespoon of oil for about 15 minutes, turning once. If making into patties, serve 2 each.

Good source of oily fish, selenium, and vitamin D. Source of **Allium** *vegetables*
PER PORTION: 304 CAL, 11.6G FAT, 2.6G SATURATED FAT

festival mackerel

This interesting dish was kindly provided by Al Crisci who is the Catering Manager at High Down Prison, Surrey. It is traditionally served with a "festival" (a deep-fried stick-shaped dough dumpling) but can equally well be served with focaccia or crusty French bread.

SERVES 4

- 1 large onion, peeled and roughly chopped
- 1 tablespoon olive oil
- ½ large green cabbage, core removed, and thinly sliced
- 16-oz. can diced tomatoes
- 2 tablespoons tomato paste
- 2 garlic cloves, chopped
- 1 teaspoon chile, or to taste
- 14 ounces smoked mackerel fillets, skinned and flaked

Gently cook the onion in the olive oil until soft but not brown. Add the cabbage and mix well. Continue cooking until the cabbage wilts. Add the tomatoes, tomato paste, garlic, chile, and about ¼ cup of water. Cook until the cabbage is tender, adding some more water if it starts to dry out. When the cabbage is cooked and most of the liquid has evaporated, stir in the flaked mackerel and continue to heat until the mackerel is hot. Add some salt and pepper at the end if needed.

Good source of cruciferous vegetables, oily fish, and vitamin D. Source of Allium vegetables, lycopene, selenium, and vitamin E
PER PORTION: 463 CAL, 35.8G FAT, 6.8G SATURATED FAT

deviled mackerel with mint and tomato salad

This dish was kindly provided by John Walter, Head Chef at the University of Surrey's Lakeside Restaurant. The fresh tangy salad carries off the spices and oily fish beautifully.

SERVES 4

- pinch of cayenne pepper
- 1 teaspoon paprika
- 1 teaspoon ground coriander
- 1 teaspoon finely ground black pepper
- 1 teaspoon English mustard powder
- 1 teaspoon sugar
- salt
- 3 tablespoons olive oil
- 2 tablespoons red wine vinegar
- 1¼–1½ pounds mackerel fillets

For the Salad
- 2 beefsteak tomatoes, chopped
- 1 small red onion, peeled and thinly sliced
- handful of fresh mint leaves
- juice of 1 lemon

Preheat the broiler to hot. Mix the spices, mustard powder, sugar, and a little salt with the olive oil and red wine vinegar.

Carefully remove any remaining bones from the mackerel fillets and, with a sharp knife, make three shallow incisions across the skin running down each fillet. Brush the fillets on both sides with the devil marinade and place on a baking tray. Place under a hot broiler for about 5 minutes until nicely browned.

To make the salad, combine the tomatoes, onion, and mint leaves in a bowl, and squeeze the lemon juice over them. To serve, pile the salad onto a plate and place the mackerel on top.

Good source of oily fish, selenium, and vitamin D. Source of lycopene
PER PORTION: 476 CAL, 36.4G FAT, 6.8G SATURATED FAT

spicy sardines with chickpea and avocado salad

This recipe was kindly provided by TV Chef Antony Worrall Thompson. This lovely salad is full of flavor and works perfectly with the oily fish.

SERVES 4

For the Chickpea and Avocado Salad
- yolk of 1 hard-boiled egg, pressed through a strainer
- ¼ cup olive oil
- 2 tablespoons red wine vinegar
- ½ red onion, finely chopped
- 1 garlic clove, crushed
- 2 tablespoons flat-leaf parsley, chopped
- 1 tablespoon small capers, drained and rinsed
- 15-oz. can chickpeas, drained and rinsed
- 1 ripe avocado, peeled and chopped into chunky cubes
- salt and ground black pepper

For the Sardines
- 1¾ tablespoons olive oil spread
- 1 fresh red chile, chopped
- 2 shallots, chopped
- 1 tablespoon flat-leaf parsley, finely chopped
- 1 tablespoon cilantro, finely chopped
- 3 garlic cloves, crushed with a little salt
- 1 tablespoon extra virgin olive oil, plus a little extra for drizzling
- 8 fresh sardines, cleaned, flattened out, backbone removed, and washed thoroughly
- juice of 1 lemon

Preheat the oven to 350°F.

To make the salad, place the egg yolk in a bowl, beat in the oil and vinegar, and stir in the onion, garlic, parsley, capers, chickpeas, and avocado, then season to taste with salt and pepper.

To cook the sardines, heat the olive oil spread in a small pan, add the chile and shallots, and cook until softened but not colored. Fold in the parsley, cilantro, garlic, and olive oil; season to taste with salt and pepper. Spread the mixture over the flesh side of the fish. Roll up the sardines and secure with 2 small wooden toothpicks, (be sure to soak the cocktail sticks in water first, to stop them from burning). Place in the oven and cook for 5–8 minutes. Drizzle with oil and lemon juice and serve two sardine rolls on a pile of salad on each plate.

Good source of Allium vegetables and legumes. Source of oily fish, selenium, vitamin D, and vitamin E
PER PORTION: 474 CAL, 39.8G FAT, 7.3G SATURATED FAT

shrimp in spicy tomato sauce (kimroun bi tamatem)

These shrimp are deliciously rich in flavor and are good hot or cold. Serve them with mashed potatoes or with a little couscous moistened with olive oil. This dish has been selected from *Arabesque* by Claudia Roden.

Use raw jumbo shrimp: they are gray and turn pink when they are cooked. Some supermarkets sell them fresh and ready-peeled. You can also buy them frozen with their heads removed. The weight of these packs is inclusive of a thick ice glaze which means that you need double the weight—i.e., for 1 pound peeled shrimp (about 25), you need a 2-pound pack.

SERVES 6

- 1 pound raw jumbo shrimp, peeled, or 2-pound pack frozen shrimp
- 1 medium onion, chopped
- 2 tablespoons extra virgin olive oil
- 3 garlic cloves, finely chopped
- 14 ounces tomatoes, peeled and chopped
- half a teaspoon ground ginger
- pinch of saffron threads (optional)
- pinch of chile pepper
- salt
- bunch of flat-leaf parsley, chopped
- bunch of cilantro, chopped

If using frozen shrimp, defrost them thoroughly. Pull the legs off the shrimp, then peel off the shells and pull off the tails (they are usually sold headless). If you see a dark thread along the back, make a fine slit with a pointed knife and pull it out.

In a large frying pan, heat the onion in the oil, stirring, until it begins to color. Add the garlic and cook until it begins to color. Then add the tomatoes, ginger, saffron (if using), chile pepper and some salt, and cook for about 20 minutes until the sauce is reduced. Now put in the shrimp and cook them for 3–5 minutes, until they turn pink, turning them over once. Stir in the cilantro and parsley at the end.

Source of Allium vegetables, lycopene, selenium, and vitamin E
PER PORTION: 125 CAL, 5.0G FAT, 0.7G SATURATED FAT

trout and leek paupiette in carrot and coriander sauce

This dish was kindly provided by John Walter, Head Chef at the University of Surrey's Lakeside Restaurant. Serve with green beans and new potatoes for a lovely, light evening meal.

SERVES 4

For the Fish
- 1 medium leek, cut in half lengthways to form strips
- ½ teaspoon each of dry-roasted and ground fennel seeds, white peppercorns, and sea salt (or Kosher salt)
- 4 skinless trout fillets

For the Sauce
- 1 shallot, finely chopped
- 1 teaspoon olive oil
- ½ teaspoon dry-roasted and ground coriander seeds
- 1 large carrot, peeled and finely grated
- scant ½ cup clear fish stock

Preheat the oven to 400°F. Plunge the leek strips into a large saucepan of boiling water and blanch for 2–3 minutes. Drain the leek strips well and divide them into four equal portions. Lay the strips of one leek portion flat on a cutting board and spread it out to about the width of one trout fillet.

Combine the trout seasoning ingredients and sprinkle them over the trout fillets. Place one seasoned trout fillet on top of the leeks and roll up from end to end. Secure the paupiette with a toothpick and place on a lightly oiled baking tray. Repeat this process with each fish and then bake for 10 minutes.

While the trout is cooking, prepare the sauce. In a saucepan, sweat the shallots in the olive oil with the coriander seeds until soft. Add the carrot and sweat for another 5 minutes. Pour over the fish stock and blend to a purée. Warm the sauce and season to taste with salt and pepper. To serve, cut each trout and leek paupiette in two and serve on a pool of carrot sauce.

Good source of oily fish and vitamin D. Source of Allium *vegetables and selenium*
PER PORTION: 227 CAL, 8.9G FAT, 2.0G SATURATED FAT

sea bream (porgy) with sun-dried tomatoes and basil

This recipe was kindly provided by TV chef Alex Mackay. Here's what Alex has to say about it:

"Braising is an excellent way to cook fish, just as healthy as poaching or steaming but much more flavorsome. In this recipe the sea bream has a quick and delightful exchange with the tomato sauce and olive oil, a process that makes everything tastier."

SERVES 4

- 1 medium onion, peeled and chopped
- 4 garlic cloves, peeled and sliced
- 3 strips of orange zest (removed with a vegetable peeler)
- 1 pound very ripe plum tomatoes, cored and roughly chopped, or 14-oz can chopped tomatoes in juice
- 3 tablespoons and 4 teaspoons extra virgin olive oil
- 2 tablespoons tomato paste
- 20 sun-dried tomatoes
- 4 large fillets of sea bream (porgy), skin on, scaled
- 1-ounce bunch of basil, leaves picked and sliced
- salt, cayenne pepper, and brown sugar

Preheat the oven to 375°F. In a covered saucepan, cook the onion, garlic, and orange peel in the 3 tablespoons of olive oil over medium heat until soft, stirring occasionally.

Add the chopped tomatoes and tomato paste along with 3 tablespoons water. Bring to a boil and simmer for 15 minutes. Discard the orange zest and season with salt, cayenne, and sugar. Add ¼ cup water and the sunblush tomatoes. Bring to a boil, then transfer the sauce to a shallow ovenproof dish large enough to hold the fish with a little space around the sides. Season the sea bream and spoon a little sauce, followed by one teaspoon of olive oil, over each fillet. Cover with baking parchment or foil and braise in the oven for 6 minutes.

Turn off the oven, leave the door ajar, and rest the sea bream for 3–4 minutes. Then plate up the sea bream, add the basil to the sauce, season to taste and spoon around the fish for serving.

Good source of Allium *vegetables, lycopene, and selenium. Source of vitamin E*
PER PORTION: 316 CAL, 27.3G FAT, 3.6G SATURATED FAT

fettuccine with salmon, zucchini, and almonds

Freshly cooked pasta served with a salmon and zucchini sauce and topped with toasted almonds is a delicious and nutritious meal. It could be accompanied by a mixed dark-green leafy salad. This dish has been adapted from a recipe in *Body and Beauty Foods* by Hazel Courteney and Kathryn Marsden.

SERVES 4

- 1¾ tablespoons olive oil spread
- ½ pound leeks, washed and thinly sliced
- ½ pound zucchini, thinly sliced
- 3 tablespoons wholewheat flour
- 1¾ cups vegetable stock
- ⅔ cup dry white wine
- 14-oz. can salmon in water, drained and flaked
- 1–2 tablespoons fresh tarragon, chopped
- dash of Tabasco sauce
- salt and freshly ground black pepper
- 12 ounces fettucine
- ⅔ cup slivered almonds, toasted
- fresh tarragon sprigs, for garnishing (or fresh parsley)

Melt the olive oil spread in a saucepan and add the leeks and zucchini. Cover and cook gently for about 10 minutes, until softened, stirring occasionally.

Add the flour and cook for 1 minute, stirring. Gradually stir in the stock and wine, then bring slowly to a boil, stirring continuously until the sauce thickens. Simmer gently for 2 minutes, stirring.

Stir the salmon, chopped tarragon, Tabasco sauce, and salt and pepper into the sauce. Reheat gently until piping hot, stirring. Meanwhile, cook the pasta in a large pot of lightly salted, boiling water until *al dente*. Drain the pasta well and transfer to serving plates. Spoon the sauce over the pasta and scatter with the almonds. Garnish with the tarragon sprigs.

Good source of vitamin D. Source of Allium *vegetables, oily fish, selenium, and vitamin E*
PER PORTION: 616 CAL, 19.5G FAT, 2.7G SATURATED FAT

poached salmon steak on spinach and watercress puree

This recipe was kindly provided by chef Raymond Blanc's kitchen. This lovely dish utilizes the technique of poaching. The salmon could be replaced by steelhead trout, flounder, or halibut. The stock can be made well in advance and the puree can be prepared 1 hour before you need it and left covered at room temperature.

SERVES 4

- 4 salmon steaks (6 ounces each)

For the Vegetable Stock
- 1 medium carrot, peeled and sliced
- 1 small onion, peeled and sliced
- 2 sticks celery, washed and chopped
- ½ medium leek, washed and sliced
- 1 strip lemon zest
- bouquet garni (2 sprigs thyme, 1 sprig parsley, 1 bay leaf, tied)
- 1 garlic clove
- 1 tablespoon sea salt (or kosher salt)
- 1 teaspoon black peppercorns
- 5 cups water, cold
- 1 cup white wine, boiled for 2 minutes

For the Spinach and Watercress Puree
- 1 tablespoon olive oil
- 7 ounces baby spinach, washed, drained, and roughly chopped
- 11½ ounces watercress, washed, drained and roughly chopped
- 2 pinches of sea salt (or kosher salt)
- pinch of black pepper, freshly ground
- 3 tablespoons soy cream

For the Lemon Sabayon
- 3 egg yolks, medium
- ¼ cup cold water
- 2 tablespoons olive oil
- pinch of sea salt (or kosher salt)
- pinch of cayenne pepper
- 2 teaspoons lemon juice

In a large pot over a high heat add all the ingredients for the stock. Boil, skim, reduce the heat, and simmer for 20 minutes.

To make the puree, heat the oil in a large pan over medium heat and add the spinach and watercress. Season with the salt and pepper and cook for 3 minutes, covered. Add the cream, bring to a boil, and simmer for another minute. Pour the mixture into a food processor and pulse for about 10 seconds until a rough texture is achieved. Taste and adjust the seasoning if needed. Place in a hot serving dish, cover, and set aside.

To cook the lemon sabayon, fill the bottom of a double boiler one-third full with water and bring to a boil. In the top pan of the double boiler, place the egg yolks and water and whisk vigorously for about 5 minutes, until you obtain a light and lemon-colored foam, about 6 or 7 times its original volume. Continue whisking until the foam has more texture but is still thin enough to run.

Pour the olive oil into the sabayon, whisk briefly. Season with salt, cayenne pepper, and lemon juice. Taste and adjust the seasoning if necessary.

To cook the salmon steaks, slide them into the simmering stock. Bring the pot back to a gentle simmer and cook the fish for 5 minutes. Turn off the heat and leave the salmon for another 2–3 minutes.

To serve, spoon the spinach and watercress puree into the middle of your plates, add the poached salmon and some of the poached vegetables on top, and generously spoon the sauce on and around the fish.

Good source of Allium vegetables, cruciferous vegetables, oily fish, selenium, and vitamin D. Source of vitamin E
PER PORTION: 549 CAL, 37.1G FAT, 6.6G SATURATED FAT

saag aloo with oily fish

This dish was kindly provided by TV chef and restaurateur Cyrus Todiwala. Here is what he has to say about it:

"This dish can be prepared with deep-fried potatoes in place of the boiled ones. Simply blanch the potatoes first, deep-fry until golden, drain well, and add at the very end. Fenugreek gives a very good flavor to this dish. It is available packaged and is known as "kasoori methi." It needs to be placed in a tray in a very slow oven until it develops a beautiful aroma. It is then crushed and sifted for tiny twigs, etc., and used in its powdered form, to flavor spinach and other dishes. To provide extra selenium, you can replace the oily fish with shrimp or chopped liver and kidney. They work extremely well with this, too, and can be stirred into the Saag Aloo before serving."

SERVES 6–8

For the Saag Aloo
- 1 pound, 10 ounces baby potatoes or ordinary ones, cubed
- 10–12 bunches of fresh spinach or 2¼ pounds picked leaves or chopped frozen spinach
- 3 tablespoons canola oil
- 1½ tablespoons cumin seeds
- 2 dried red chiles, broken into pieces
- 2 tablespoons fresh ginger, chopped
- 3 tablespoons garlic, finely chopped
- salt and crushed black pepper
- dried fenugreek, optional, for taste
- 1 large tablespoon fresh cilantro, chopped

For the Fish
- 4–5 ounces oily fish per person —fresh tuna, or swordfish will all work well
- ground turmeric, about 1 teaspoon for every 10 ounces fish
- lime juice, 1 lime for every 10 ounces fish
- a little canola oil for cooking

To prepare the fish, marinate in the turmeric and lime juice.

Boil the potatoes until soft but still firm. Blanch the spinach briefly in boiling water, taking care not to overcook it; drain, and either finely chop or puree. If pureeing the spinach, there may be no need to blanch in water as the spinach will contain a great deal of water and will wilt down in a dry saucepan.

Heat the oil in a deep pot or a frying pan large enough to hold all the potato and the spinach—a wok would be ideal. Add the cumin and red chile pieces and cook for about half a minute or so. Add the chopped ginger and garlic and continue cooking.

As the garlic begins to turn a deep golden color add the spinach and sauté for a few minutes stirring regularly. Add salt and crushed pepper to taste, and dried crumbled fenugreek if using. Stir in the potatoes and simmer for a minute or two until they are heated through. Stir in the fresh chopped cilantro for the final touch.

Brush the fish with a little oil and cook under the broiler or in a frying pan on the stove for a few minutes until the flesh flakes. Slice the fish and place it on the Saag Aloo for serving.

Good source of oily fish and vitamin D. Source of Allium *vegetables, selenium, and vitamin E.*
PER PORTION: 393 CAL, 20.6G FAT, 3.4G SATURATED FAT

POM stuffed halibut

This fish dish can be served with rice and fresh green vegetables such as peas or beans. Other fish can be used—just make sure that the fillets are thin enough to roll. This dish has been adapted from a recipe on www.pomwonderful.com.

SERVES 4

- 1¼ pounds halibut fillets, ⅝-inch thick
- 1 teaspoon salt
- 3 tablespoons olive oil
- 1 onion, thinly sliced
- 3 garlic cloves, crushed
- ¼ teaspoon freshly ground black pepper
- ⅓ cup chopped walnuts
- 1 tablespoon slivered candied orange peel

- 1 cup pomegranate juice
- ¼ teaspoon ground saffron, dissolved in 2 tablespoons hot water
- 2 tablespoons fresh lime juice

For the Garnish
- 2 tablespoons chopped walnuts
- 2 tablespoons pomegranate arils

Preheat the oven to 400°F.

Rinse the fish in cold water, pat dry with paper towels, and rub both sides with salt and set aside.

Heat 2 tablespoons of oil in a large frying pan and brown the onion and garlic. Add the pepper, walnuts, candied peel, and pomegranate juice, and cook for 3 minutes. Mix well and remove from the heat.

Lay the fish out on a baking dish and place a quarter of the fried stuffing on one end of each of the fish fillets. Gently roll the fish from the stuffing end and pin closed with a toothpick, if necessary. Pour the saffron water, the remaining oil, and the lime juice over the fish.

Place in the oven and bake for 10–15 minutes, basting from time to time, until the fish flakes easily with a fork. Arrange the fish on a serving platter. Pour the sauce from the baking dish over the fish and garnish with walnuts and pomegranate arils.

Good source of Allium *vegetables and selenium. Source of polyphenols and vitamin E*
PER PORTION: 454 CAL, 27.2G FAT, 3.1G SATURATED FAT

liver and onions

This rich and traditional meal is great comfort food served on a mound of mashed potatoes. This recipe has been selected from *Cooking with the Kosher Butcher's Wife* by Sharon Lurie.

SERVES 4–5

- 18 ounces calf's or ox's liver, sliced
- ½ cup flour
- 3 large onions, cut in half and sliced into half rounds
- a little olive oil for frying
- ½ teaspoon freshly crushed garlic

- ¼ cup red wine (optional)
- ½ cup chicken stock (either homemade or ½ chicken bouillon cube dissolved in 1 cup hot water)
- freshly ground black pepper (optional)

Cut the liver into the size pieces you'd like and coat with the flour. Cook the onions in oil until glassy, then add the garlic and toss for a minute or two.

Add the liver to the onions and continue frying over medium heat or until the onions are golden brown. Don't let the pan burn as this will give the gravy a bitter taste.

Add the wine, if using, and add the chicken stock, stirring as you do so to get all the bits off the bottom of the pan. This, together with the onions, gives the gravy its delicious taste. Let the gravy thicken and reduce slightly.

If you feel your gravy is too thick, add a little more water and bring to a boil. Add salt and freshly ground black pepper.

Good source of Allium *vegetables and selenium*
PER PORTION: 331 CAL, 11.6G FAT, 2.2G SATURATED FAT

moroccan lamb stew

This is a fragrant stew with a Moroccan vibe. Don't let the number of ingredients put you off—the oven does the hard work!

SERVES 6

- 3 tablespoons olive oil
- 1 large onion, finely chopped
- 1 tablespoon ground cumin
- 1 tablespoon ground cinnamon
- 2 teaspoons turmeric
- black pepper
- 5 garlic cloves, finely chopped
- 1½ pounds lamb, trimmed of fat and chopped into ¾-inch cubes
- 2 x 16-oz. cans chopped tomatoes
- 3 tablespoons tomato paste
- 7 ounces carrots, cut into sticks
- 14 ounces parsnips, chopped into sticks

- ½ cup dried apricots, roughly chopped
- ½ cup golden raisins
- 2½ cups lamb or chicken stock
- 15-ounce can chickpeas
- small bunch of fresh cilantro, chopped
- ⅔ cup lowfat yogurt or soy yogurt

For the Couscous
- 2¼ cups couscous
- 1 tablespoon mint sauce or chopped fresh mint
- 3½ ounces pomegranate arils

Preheat the oven to 300°F.

Heat 2 tablespoons of the oil in a large flameproof and ovenproof pan and gently cook the onion and spices for 10 minutes, adding the garlic for the last 3 minutes.

Meanwhile, in a separate pan, cook the lamb in the remaining tablespoon of oil for 8 minutes. Transfer the lamb to the onion and stir in the chopped tomatoes, tomato paste, chopped vegetables, dried fruits, and stock. Bring to a boil, cover, and put in the oven for 2 hours. Stir in the chickpeas for the second hour.

Ten minutes before the stew is ready, stir the mint into the couscous and cook according to package instructions. When the couscous is ready, fluff it up with a fork and stir in the pomegranate arils. Serve the stew and couscous with a little yogurt and the chopped cilantro sprinkled on top.

Good source of Allium *vegetables and lycopene. Source of legumes and vitamin E*
PER PORTION: 619 CAL, 20.1G FAT, 5.8G SATURATED FAT

beef and lentil cottage pie

This provides a hearty meal full of flavor. Using lentils gives the benefit of legumes while reducing the quantity of red meat. Serve on its own or with vegetables.

SERVES 4

- ½ pound lean ground beef
- 1 large onion
- ¾ cup green lentils, rinsed
- 16-oz. can diced tomatoes
- 4 carrots, peeled and chopped
- 1¼ cups frozen peas
- ¾ cup beef or vegetable stock
- 2 tablespoons tomato ketchup

For the Mashed Potato Topping
- 2¼ pounds potatoes, peeled and chopped
- 1¾ tablespoons olive oil spread
- 2–3 tablespoons milk or soy milk

Preheat the oven to 350°F.

Put the beef and onions in a large pan and cook until the beef has browned. Add the remaining ingredients and cook for about 30 minutes, until the lentils and vegetables are soft, adding a little water if necessary. Pour into an ovenproof dish.

Meanwhile, boil the potatoes until tender. Drain and mash them, adding the olive oil spread and enough milk to make a soft mash. Scoop the potatoes on top of the beef mixture and place in the oven for 30 minutes or until the top is golden brown.

Good source of selenium. Source of Allium *vegetables, lycopene, and legumes*
PER PORTION: 541 CAL, 11.8G FAT, 3.2G SATURATED FAT

small meats (laham saghir)

This recipe was picked up by Granny Dilley during her years in Yemen and she doubts there is a formal recipe for it. It owes a lot to the old trading contacts between Yemen, Indonesia, and India. It is traditional to add a good amount of finely chopped garlic lightly stirred in or sprinkled on top just before serving—but you can add it all at the beginning. Serve with French bread or rice and "Chop-it-up" (page 147). This recipe has been kindly provided by Mrs. John Dilley.

SERVES 2

- 1 tablespoon soy oil
- 1 medium onion, quite finely chopped
- 3–4 garlic cloves, finely chopped
- 2 teaspoons curry powder or paste (Hot Madras)
- 2 teaspoons ground cumin
- 1 chile (Thai bird's eye), chopped with seeds (or more, to taste)
- 2 teaspoons ground coriander
- 1 small–medium waxy potato, cut into ½-inch cubes (optional)
- ½ pound lambs' liver and/or kidneys, coarsely chopped
- 1 tablespoon tomato paste
- 16-oz. can diced tomatoes
- sea salt (or kosher salt) and ground black pepper

Heat the oil in a frying pan over medium heat and lightly cook the onion, garlic, spices, chile, and potato (if using) for about 10 minutes. Stir occasionally and do not let it burn; add a little extra oil if necessary.

Add the "small meats," tomato paste and diced tomatoes, swirl a little water around the inside of the can, and pour into the pan. Season with salt and pepper. Cook over medium–high heat for 5–10 minutes or until cooked through and the sauce has the degree of thickness you like, stirring occasionally. Serve hot or cold. This dish improves with keeping and can be made a day in advance.

Good source of Allium vegetables, lycopene, and selenium. Source of vitamin E
PER PORTION: 332 CAL, 14.2G FAT, 2.5G SATURATED FAT

dr. john's meatballs

This is a satisfying dish of succulent meatballs in a deliciously rich sauce. To reduce the amount of meat, simply replace ½ pound of the ground steak with 8 ounces tofu that has been mashed with a fork, and crumble in two beef bouillion cubes. Small new potatoes can be added to the casserole for the last 30–40 minutes of cooking.

SERVES 4

- 2¼ pounds onions
- 2 tablespoons olive oil
- 2 teaspoons cornflour
- salt and pepper

For the Meatballs
- 18 ounces ground steak
- 1 medium egg, beaten
- 1 teaspoon horseradish, or more to taste
- salt and pepper
- 1 tablespoon flour
- 1 tablespoon olive oil

Preheat the oven to 350°F.

Finely slice the onions and sweat gently in the olive oil in an iron casserole until they are a uniform mid- to dark brown. Mix the cornstarch with a little cold water in a measuring cup and then add boiling water to the mixture to make up to 2½ cups. Add the cornstarch and water mixture to the onions and stir. Add a good amount of salt and pepper and simmer very gently until you are ready to add the meatballs.

In a large bowl combine the meat, beaten egg, and horseradish and a good seasoning of salt and pepper. Add enough flour to bind the mixture (about a tablespoon). Form the meat mixture into small balls about the size of a golf ball.

Cook gently in a frying pan in 1 tablespoon of olive oil, until they are browned all over. Remove from the pan and drain on paper towels. Put the meatballs into the simmering sauce, cover tightly, and cook in a moderate oven for 1½ hours or until the meatballs are tender, adding a little more water if necessary. Adjust seasoning before serving.

Good source of Allium *vegetables. Source of selenium*
PER PORTION: 479 CAL, 29.0G FAT, 10.3G SATURATED FAT

stir-fried pork tenderloin

There are numerous ways you could vary this tasty stir-fry: you could use chicken breast instead of pork, add a tablespoon of fish sauce in with the soy sauce, or add peanuts or cashews. Why not try some of the following as alternative or additional vegetables: zucchini, snow peas, canned water chestnuts, canned bamboo shoots, or mushrooms.

SERVES 4

For the Pork and Marinade
- 2 tablespoons soy sauce, plus extra to taste
- 1 tablespoon lemon juice
- 1 teaspoon brown sugar
- 1 pork tenderloin, cut into thin strips

For the Vegetable Stir-fry
- 2 tablespoons canola oil
- 1 inch fresh ginger, grated
- 2 garlic cloves, chopped

- 1 red chile, seeded and chopped
- 1 red onion, thinly sliced
- 1 head of broccoli, broken into small florets
- 1 bok choy, sliced
- 1 bunch of scallions, chopped into ½ inch pieces
- 11 ounces bean sprouts
- 1 each of red, green, and yellow peppers, sliced into thin strips
- salt

Combine the marinade ingredients in a bowl and add the pork strips. Leave in the fridge to marinate for at least 2 hours, or ideally overnight.

Drain the meat from the marinade and pat dry with paper towels. Heat the oil in a large wok. When the oil is just smoking, stir-fry the ginger, garlic, and chile for 10–20 seconds and then add the pork. Stir-fry the pork until lightly browned, then add the red onion and broccoli, and stir-fry for another minute. Add the remaining vegetables and continue to stir-fry for 4–5 minutes more.

Add the marinade from the meat and a little more soy sauce to taste, and cook for another 2 minutes. Season with salt and serve with boiled rice.

Good source of Allium *vegetables, cruciferous vegetables, and legumes*
PER PORTION: 223 CAL, 9.9G FAT, 1.3G SATURATED FAT

badak chaanti badami pasanda (stuffed duck breast in a creamy sauce)

This dish has been kindly provided by TV chef and restaurateur Cyrus Todiwala. This is what he has to say about it:

"The sauce is a version of korma and can be used with any other meat, fish, poultry, or vegetables. The word pasanda *represents the stuffing and relates to any form of stuffing. Badami* stands for *with or of almonds."*

This recipe uses ginger and garlic paste which is very easy to make. Simply blend together equal quantities of garlic and fresh ginger with a little oil and water until a smooth puree is formed.

This paste can be kept in the fridge for up to six months in an airtight jar.

SERVES 6

- 6 medium-sized duck breasts

For the Stuffing
- ⅔ cup ricotta or paneer
- 6–8 whole almonds, sliced or coarsely chopped
- 6–8 Brazil nuts, sliced or coarsely chopped, plus extra for garnishing
- 10–15 golden raisins
- generous pinch of ground cardamom
- salt, to taste
- 1 tablespoon chopped fresh cilantro
- a few threads saffron (a small pinch will give you the desired number of threads)

For the Sauce
- 2 tablespoons canola oil
- 2 medium onions, sliced
- 1 tablespoon ginger and garlic paste
- ¼ teaspoon turmeric
- ½ teaspoon ground cumin
- ¾ teaspoon ground coriander
- ½ teaspoon chile powder
- 1 cup ground almonds
- 1 cup cashews

For the Tempering
- 1 tablespoon canola oil
- 1-inch piece cinnamon
- 3–4 cardamom pods
- 3 cloves
- 2 peppercorns
- 1 mace flower, broken into two
- 1–2 bay leaves

Blend all the stuffing ingredients together, season to taste with salt and pepper, and set aside in the refrigerator to keep firm.

Trim some of the skin and fat from the duck breasts but do not remove it all. With a thin, sharp knife, slit the duck breasts through the middle and carefully open them out, taking care not to pierce the meat or separate it completely. With gentle, short strokes, the meat should separate fairly easily and cleanly. Open the duck breasts out and lay them out in a row.

Spoon equal quantities of the stuffing onto one edge of each of the open duck breasts, fold the edge over the stuffing, and roll up until you have a sausage. Once rolled, wrap each duck breast in a piece of aluminum foil. Place them in a large pan deep enough to fit them all. Pour in enough hot or boiling water to cover, and simmer for about 20 minutes. Let the duck breasts cool in the liquid. When cold, skim off any fat and retain the stock for the sauce.

To cook the sauce, heat the oil in a large pan. Add the onions and sauté for 5–6 minutes or until opaque. Add the ginger and garlic paste and all the spices, and sauté for 2–3 minutes. Next add the ground almonds and cashews and sauté for 4–5 minutes, stirring with a wooden spatula but do not let them burn. Add about 1 cup of the reserved stock and stir. If the mixture gets too thick, add some more stock. Boil gently for 15 minutes or until the onions and cashews are cooked. If the sauce thickens too much, add a little more stock. Cool the sauce and puree in the blender. Reheat the sauce and bring to a slow boil, stirring regularly.

Heat the oil for the tempering and fry the spices. When they are browned and swollen, put them into the sauce, stir well, and season to taste with salt and pepper. To serve, remove the duck breasts from the foil, clean the sides with paper towels and place them in the hot sauce. Continue to heat the sauce very gently until the duck breasts are thoroughly reheated. Slice the duck breasts and serve on a platter with the sauce poured on top. Garnish with some extra slivers of Brazil nuts.

Good source of Allium vegetables and selenium. Source of vitamin E
PER PORTION: 584 CAL, 39.2G FAT, 7.6G SATURATED FAT

stuffed eggplant (karniyarik)

These eggplants stuffed with ground meat are served as a hot main dish with rice pilaf. Use small, elongated eggplants (at most 5½ inches long), weighing about 4½ ounces. This dish has been selected from *Arabesque* by Claudia Roden.

SERVES 6

- 6 thin and long medium-sized eggplants
- 1 tablespoon salt
- 2–3 tablespoons sunflower oil
- 2 onions, chopped
- 14 ounces ground beef or lamb
- 1 tablespoon tomato paste
- 2 large tomatoes, peeled and chopped
- 1 teaspoon ground cinnamon
- ½ teaspoon ground allspice
- salt and black pepper
- large bunch of flat-leaf parsley, chopped
- 1 cup tomato juice

Preheat the oven to 350°F.

Trim the caps but leave the stems on the eggplants. Peel ¾-inch strips off the skins lengthways, leaving ¾-inch strips of peel. Soak the eggplants in water mixed with 1 tablespoon of salt for 30 minutes, then drain and dry. Fry 2–3 at a time very briefly in hot shallow oil, turning to brown them lightly all over. Drain on paper towels.

For the filling, cook the onions in another pan in 2–3 tablespoons oil until soft. Add the meat and cook for about 10 minutes. Add the tomato paste and one of the tomatoes, plus the spices, salt and pepper. Stir well and simmer until the liquid is reduced.

Place the eggplants side by side in a single layer in an ovenproof dish. With a sharp pointed knife, make a slit in each one, lengthways, along one of the skinless strips on the top until about an inch from each end. Carefully open the slits and, with a spoon, press against the flesh on the insides to make a hollow pocket. Fill each of the eggplants with the filling, and place a slice of the remaining tomato on top. Pour the tomato juice into the dish, cover with foil, and bake in the oven for about 40 minutes or until the eggplants are soft.

Good source of lycopene. Source of Allium vegetables and vitamin E
PER PORTION: 265 CAL, 16.5G FAT, 5.6G SATURATED FAT

chicken cobbler

This chicken cobbler makes a hearty mid-week meal. You could substitute 1¼ cups of the chicken stock with white wine if you like.

SERVES 4

- 18 ounces skinless chicken breast, diced
- 1 tablespoon flour
- 2 tablespoons canola oil
- 2 medium leeks, sliced
- 2 cups frozen fava beans
- 11 ounces carrots, peeled and sliced or chopped
- 2 celery sticks, sliced
- 2½ cups chicken stock

For the Scone Topping
- 1¾ cups flour
- 1 tablespoon baking powder
- ½ teaspoon salt
- 1¾ tablespoons olive oil spread
- 1 tablespoon sunflower seeds
- 1 egg, beaten
- water for mixing

Preheat the oven to 350°F.

Toss the chopped chicken breast in the flour until it is coated. Heat the oil in a flameproof and ovenproof pan, add the chicken pieces, and cook, stirring until the meat has sealed. Add the vegetables and cook, stirring for another 2–3 minutes. Add the stock and bring to a boil. Cover the pan and place in the oven for about 1 hour.

Towards the end of the cooking time, check the dish and add some water if necessary. Meanwhile, make the scone topping. Sift the flour and baking powder into a bowl and add the salt. Rub in the olive oil spread until the mixture resembles fine breadcrumbs. Stir in the sunflower seeds and then the egg and about 2–3 tablespoons of water to form a soft dough. Divide the mixture into 8 equal portions and roll into balls.

When the chicken dish has cooked for an hour, remove it from the oven and place the scone balls on top. Brush the scones with any remaining beaten egg or a little milk. Return to the oven, uncovered, for 20–30 minutes or until the scones are golden brown.

Source of Allium vegetables, legumes, selenium, and vitamin E
PER PORTION: 548 CAL, 14.9G FAT, 2.5G SATURATED FAT

chicken kebabs with peanut sauce

You can substitute the chicken with pork or beef tenderloin. Serve with plain boiled rice and Broccoli Saltati (page 153). The peanut sauce will freeze very well. This recipe has been kindly provided by Dr John Rayman.

SERVES 4

- 4 chicken breasts, sliced into thick strips

For the Marinade
- 3 tablespoons soy sauce
- 1 tablespoon lemon juice
- 1 tablespoon olive oil
- 1 medium onion, chopped
- 3 garlic cloves, chopped
- 1 teaspoon chile powder
- 1-inch piece fresh ginger, grated
- 2 teaspoons brown sugar

For the Peanut Sauce
- ½ teaspoon turmeric
- ½ teaspoon curry powder
- ½ teaspoon cayenne pepper
- 2 teaspoons sugar
- 1 cup coconut milk
- 1 cup salted peanuts, coarsely ground
- 1 teaspoon lemon juice, or to taste
- salt

Mix all the marinade ingredients together in a bowl and add the chicken, ensuring that all the pieces are covered. Let it marinate in the fridge for 24 hours.

Preheat the oven to 400°F.

To make the sauce, combine the turmeric, curry powder, cayenne pepper, sugar, and coconut milk in a saucepan, and bring gently to a boil. Stirring constantly, add the peanuts and simmer for 2–3 minutes or until the sauce has thickened. Add lemon juice and salt to taste. You may need to add a little more coconut milk if the sauce becomes too thick.

Thread the strips of chicken onto skewers and place on a baking tray. Cook in the oven for 25–30 minutes or until the chicken is cooked through, basting with the marinade occasionally. Serve with the peanut sauce.

Good source of Allium vegetables. Source of selenium, legumes
PER PORTION: 476 CAL, 20.6G FAT, 4.0G SATURATED FAT

thai green curry

This is a fragrant, Asian curry which can be served in bowls with rice and soy sauce. This recipe has been kindly provided by Sarah Dilley.

SERVES 4

- 1 tablespoon flavorless oil or nut oil
- ¼ cup Thai green curry paste
- 4 chicken breasts, cubed
- 1 carrot, sliced into rounds
- 1 pepper, sliced
- 5½ ounces frozen soybeans (edamame)
- 1½ ounces green beans
- ¾ pound broccoli
- 16-oz can coconut milk
- 1 tablespoon fish sauce
- small bunch of fresh cilantro, chopped
- lime wedges, for serving

Heat the oil in a wok or large frying pan over medium–high heat. Add the Thai green curry paste and cook, stirring, for 2 minutes.

Add the chicken breasts and stir-fry for 5 minutes, then add all the vegetables to the pan and stir-fry for 3 minutes more.

Pour in the coconut milk and fish sauce and let it simmer for 5–10 minutes, stirring occasionally, until the vegetables are cooked and the sauce has thickened. Stir in most of the chopped cilantro. Garnish with lime wedges and the remaining cilantro when ready to serve.

Good source of cruciferous vegetables. Source of selenium and soy
PER PORTION: 433 CAL, 13.2G FAT, 3.1G SATURATED FAT

persian rice with chicken and tomatoes

This colorful, family-pleasing dish is based on a Persian recipe. The amounts and combinations of spices can be altered according to what you have in the pantry. You could use pork or lamb in place of the chicken, and serve with a leafy salad.

SERVES 6

- 1 teaspoon turmeric
- ½ teaspoon cardamom pods
- ½ teaspoon cumin
- ½ teaspoon cinnamon
- ½ teaspoon coriander seeds
- pinch of caraway seeds
- 4 peppercorns
- 6 cloves
- 1 tablespoon olive oil
- 1 large onion, sliced
- 4 garlic cloves, finely chopped
- salt
- 1¼ pounds chicken (4 breast fillets), cut into small cubes
- 3 tablespoons tomato paste
- 2 cups long-grain rice (basmati)
- 6 ounces new potatoes (or any waxy potatoes, e.g. Maris Piper), cut into small cubes
- 18 ounces cherry tomatoes or 16-oz. can diced tomatoes
- fresh cilantro, chopped, for serving
- yogurt or soy yogurt, for serving (optional)

Grind together the spices with a mortar and pestle. Heat the oil and lightly cook the onion in a large pan for about 5 minutes. Add the garlic and continue to cook until the onion is soft and golden.

Stir in the spices and salt and cook for a minute more. Add the chicken and fry, stirring, for about 8 minutes until browned. Stir in the tomato paste, then the rice and potatoes, then the tomatoes.

Add 3½ cups boiling water, cover, and simmer over low heat for 30 minutes until the rice is cooked and has absorbed all the water. To serve, top with a little yogurt and sprinkle with fresh cilantro.

Good source of Allium *vegetables. Source of lycopene, selenium*
PER PORTION: 430 CAL, 5.2G FAT, 1.0G SATURATED FAT

chicken with walnut and pomegranate sauce

This delicious dish should be eaten with plain rice and a green salad. The recipe has been kindly provided by Dr. John Rayman.

SERVES 4

- 3 tablespoons olive oil
- 1 large onion, finely chopped
- 1 cup coarsely chopped walnuts, plus extra for garnishing
- juice of 2 oranges
- 1¾ cups pomegranate juice
- 1 teaspoon salt
- 1 teaspoon cinnamon
- 1 tablespoon sugar
- ¾ teaspoon saffron
- heaping ⅓ cup flour
- 1 teaspoon turmeric
- 1 medium chicken, skinned and cut up
- handful of pomegranate arils for serving (optional)

Cook the onion gently in 1 tablespoon of olive oil in a heavy pan until light brown in color. Add the walnuts and cook very slowly for 4 minutes, stirring continuously to prevent the mixture from burning.

Add the orange juice, pomegranate juice, salt, cinnamon, sugar, and saffron. Simmer over low heat for 2–3 minutes. Mix the flour and turmeric on a flat plate. Carefully roll each chicken piece in the mixture to cover thoroughly.

Heat 2 tablespoons of olive oil in a large frying pan and fry the chicken over low–medium heat until it is golden brown all over. Remove from the pan and drain on paper towels.

Add the chicken pieces to the walnut and pomegranate sauce and simmer for 40 minutes or until the chicken is tender and thoroughly cooked. Garnish with walnuts and pomegranate arils, if you like.

Good source of polyphenols. Source of Allium *vegetables and selenium*
PER PORTION: 614 CAL, 31.2G FAT, 4.0G SATURATED FAT

pheasant with dried shiitake mushrooms

This dish is excellent served with peas or snow peas and boiled new potatoes. It can also be made with other kinds of game such as partridge. For an additional source of selenium, if you have the livers of the pheasants, they can be added at the end of the browning stage. This dish has been kindly provided by Dr. John Rayman.

SERVES 6

- 1 ounce dried shiitake mushrooms
- 3 tablespoons olive oil
- 2 pheasants, cleaned and dried
- 1¾ cups good red wine
- 1 tablespoon flour
- 20 pearl onions

Preheat the oven to 400°F.

Soak the mushrooms in warm water according to the package instructions, then drain and reserve for later. Heat 2 tablespoons of olive oil in a heavy frying pan and cook the pheasants until fairly tender and nicely browned all over.

Remove to a heavy ovenproof dish and keep warm. Add red wine to the frying pan and bring to a boil. Reduce to half its volume, stir in the flour, and pour the sauce over the reserved birds. Season with salt and pepper. Blanch the onions in boiling salted water and dry. Heat 1 tablespoon of olive oil in a frying pan, brown the onions, and add to the pheasants.

Place in the oven and cook for 45 minutes or until the birds are tender. Towards the end of the cooking, add the soaked mushrooms to the dish. Adjust the seasoning and serve.

Good source of Allium *vegetables and vitamin D. Source of selenium*
PER PORTION: 502 CAL, 12.9G FAT, 2.7G SATURATED FAT

jardaloo ma murghi (chicken with apricots)

This dish has been kindly provided by TV chef and restaurateur Cyrus Todiwala. This is what he has to say about it:

"This is a very popular Parsee chicken preparation served at festive occasions and dates back to our Persian ancestry. This dish can be served garnished with crispy straw potatoes and accompanied with chapatis, bread, or plain rice."

SERVES 4–6

- 7 ounces dried apricots
- ¼ cup canola oil
- 2 x 1-inch pieces cinnamon stick
- 2 medium onions, chopped
- 2 heaping tablespoons ginger and garlic paste (see note on recipe, page 116)
- 1¼ pounds chicken, cut into ¾-inch pieces
- 16-oz. can diced tomatoes
- salt, to taste

- 1–2 tablespoons cilantro, chopped

For the Masala
- 6–8 large sized dry red chiles
- 1½ teaspoons cumin seeds
- 1½ tablespoons coriander seeds
- 1-inch piece cinnamon stick
- 4–5 green cardamom pods
- 4–5 cloves

Soak the apricots beforehand in about 1 cup of warm water for 2–3 hours or overnight, until they are swollen and soft. Grind the masala spices together with as little water as possible to make a thick paste and set aside.

Heat the oil in a large heavy pan until hazy and add the cinnamon sticks. After about 1½ minutes, add the onions and brown slowly. Add the masala and ginger and garlic paste, and sauté well until the absorbed oil is released slowly around the edges of the combined masala and onions. Add the chicken and sauté for 4–5 minutes.

Add salt to taste, and the diced tomatoes and the apricots, along with any water that has not been absorbed. Mix well, cover, and simmer until the chicken is cooked through. If the gravy becomes too thin, remove the lid. Blend in the chopped cilantro, then check the seasoning and serve.

Good source of** Allium **vegetables. Source of lycopene, selenium, and vitamin E
PER PORTION: 409 CAL, 17.3G FAT, 1.2G SATURATED FAT

turkey and apricot casserole

This creamy recipe is simple to make and a real family pleaser. Using soy milk rather than regular milk not only reduces the dairy content but increases the soy content. To make this dish dairy-free, simply replace the cheese with a cheese substitute. This dish has been adapted from a Sainsbury's recipe.

SERVES 4

- 1 pound turkey, cut into strips
- 3 tablespoons flour
- ground black pepper
- 1 tablespoon olive oil
- 1 cup scallions, sliced
- 1½ cups chopped dried apricots
- 1¼ cups soy milk
- ¾ cup shredded sharp cheddar cheese

For the Topping
- 1½ ounces wholewheat breadcrumbs
- ¼ cup Brazil nuts, chopped
- 2 tablespoons fresh parsley, chopped
- ¼ cup shredded sharp cheddar cheese

Preheat the oven to 375°F.

Coat the turkey strips in the flour, seasoned with pepper. Heat the oil in a nonstick pan. Add the turkey and cook for 2–3 minutes, stirring continually until sealed.

Stir in the scallions and apricots, followed by the soy milk. Cook for 2–3 minutes, stirring until thickened and smooth. Stir in ¾ cup of the cheese and transfer the mixture to an ovenproof dish. Mix together the breadcrumbs, nuts, most of the parsley, and the remaining cheese. Sprinkle this over the turkey mixture.

Bake for 15 minutes. For a crispy topping, place under a preheated broiler for 1–2 minutes. Garnish with the remaining parsley.

Good source of selenium. Source of** Allium **vegetables and soy
PER PORTION: 435 CAL, 19.2G FAT, 7.6G SATURATED FAT

sweet and sour turkey meatballs

Serve these tasty meatballs with mashed potatoes and fresh vegetables. This dish has been adapted from a recipe in *Body and Beauty Foods* by Hazel Courteney and Kathryn Marsden.

SERVES 4

- 1 pound turkey ground
- 4 shallots or 1 onion, finely chopped
- 2 garlic cloves, crushed
- 1¾ cups finely chopped mushrooms
- 2 teaspoons mixed dried herbs
- 2 ounces fresh wholewheat breadcrumbs
- 2 tablespoons tomato paste
- salt and pepper
- a little wholewheat flour
- 1 tablespoon olive oil

For the Sauce
- 1 tablespoon cornstarch
- ¼ cup red wine
- 16-oz. can diced tomatoes, pureed
- ²⁄₃ cup unsweetened apple juice
- 2 tablespoons red wine vinegar
- 2 tablespoons brown sugar
- 1 tablespoon tomato paste

Preheat the oven to 350°F.

Put all the meatball ingredients, except the flour and the oil, in a bowl and mix well. Roll the mixture into small balls. Sprinkle the flour on a plate and roll each meatball lightly in it. Place the meatballs on a plate and chill for 20 minutes.

To make the sauce, blend the cornstarch with the red wine in a saucepan. Add the remaining sauce ingredients. Bring to a boil, stirring continuously, then reduce the heat and simmer while you start cooking the meatballs.

Heat the oil in a frying pan and fry the meatballs over medium heat for 5–10 minutes, until light brown. Transfer to an ovenproof dish and pour the sauce over the meatballs. Cover and bake for about 45 minutes or until the meatballs are cooked.

Source of Allium *vegetables, lycopene, and selenium*
PER PORTION: 293 CAL, 5.5G FAT, 1.0G SATURATED FAT

falafel with tomato and cucumber relish

Falafel is a popular street food in many countries around the world. By baking it rather than deep-frying, the fat content is instantly reduced. This vegetarian classic tastes great with the tomato and cucumber relish.

SERVES 6

- 6 wholewheat pita breads
- 2 cups salad greens

For the Falafel
- 2 x 15-oz. cans chickpeas, drained
- 3 garlic cloves, peeled
- 1 large onion, chopped
- 1 teaspoon ground cumin
- ½ teaspoon ground coriander
- pinch of cayenne pepper or 1 teaspoon chile powder

- salt and pepper
- 1 cup chopped fresh parsley
- 2 tablespoons lemon juice
- 1 tablespoon olive oil

For the Tomato and Cucumber Relish
- 3 tomatoes
- ½ English cucumber
- ²⁄₃ cup soy yogurt
- 1 tablespoon mint sauce

Preheat the oven to 350°F.

Put all the falafel ingredients except the olive oil in a food processor and blend until coarse; do not let the mixture become smooth. If you have time, make the mixture in advance and chill in the fridge for a few hours for the flavors to infuse. Form small handfuls of the mixture into 12–16 balls. Wearing plastic gloves makes the falafel easier to handle as they stop it sticking to your hands.

Grease a baking tray with the olive oil and place the falafel balls on it. Bake in the oven for 30 minutes or until golden brown, turning once. To make the relish, chop the tomatoes and cucumber into small cubes of uniform size. In a bowl, mix the tomato and cucumber cubes with the soy yogurt and mint. Warm the pita breads in the oven for a few minutes, but don't let them go crispy. Serve the falafel with the pita bread, soy yogurt relish, and salad greens.

Good source of Allium *vegetables and legumes. Source of soy and vitamin E*
PER PORTION: 304 CAL, 6.9G FAT, 0.9G SATURATED FAT

spicy bean pita

These spicy bean pitas make a filling and warming lunch. This dish has been adapted from a recipe in Morrisons' supermarket magazine, *Let's Eat Smart*.

SERVES 4

- 2 tablespoons olive oil
- 8 scallions, finely chopped
- 1 red pepper, cubed
- 15-oz. can butter beans (or lima beans), drained and rinsed
- 16-oz. can diced tomatoes
- 2 tablespoons sweet chile sauce
- 4 wholewheat pita breads
- 1 bunch of watercress

Heat the oil in a small pan. Add the scallions and red pepper and sauté until tender.

Add the butter beans, tomatoes, and chile sauce and cook until the sauce thickens. Slice the pita breads in half and lightly toast, if you like.

Spoon the butter bean mixture into the pitta breads and garnish with the watercress.

Source of** Allium **vegetables, cruciferous vegetables, legumes, lycopene, and vitamin E
PER PORTION: 407 CAL, 9.0G FAT, 1.4G SATURATED FAT

bean burgers

Make these bean burgers as spicy or mild as you like by simply adding more or less chile. Serve them in a hamburger bun with ketchup and a side salad.

SERVES 4

- 1 medium potato, peeled and chopped
- 2 tablespoons oil
- 1 medium onion, finely chopped
- 3 garlic cloves, finely chopped
- 1 teaspoon cumin
- 1 teaspoon coriander
- 1 red chile or 1 teaspoon chile powder or to taste
- 8 ounces frozen soybeans (edamame)
- 15-oz. can kidney beans, drained
- small bunch of fresh cilantro
- salt and pepper
- ¼ cup corn

Boil the potato in a pan of boiling water for 15 minutes or until soft; drain and mash. Heat a tablespoon of the oil in a pan and gently cook the onion for about 3 minutes. Add the garlic and spices and cook for another 3 minutes.

In a pan of water, boil the soybeans for 5 minutes or until cooked. Drain the beans and mash all the ingredients together with a potato masher. Alternatively, you could put all the ingredients into a blender or food processor and pulse until coarse, not smooth.

Form the mixture into 8 patties, then set aside to rest for an hour or so. Heat the remaining tablespoon of oil in a nonstick frying pan and cook the bean burgers for about 5 minutes on each side.

Good source of Allium *vegetables and legumes. Source of soy*
PER PORTION: 274 CAL, 11.3G FAT, 1.7G SATURATED FAT

leek and butter bean crumble

This crumble makes for a wholesome and heart-warming meal which can be served with green leafy vegetables. This recipe has been kindly provided by Sylvia Wainwright.

SERVES 3

- 2 large leeks, sliced
- 1 garlic clove, crushed
- 4 tomatoes, roughly chopped
- 1 tablespoon canola oil
- 15-oz. can butter beans (or lima beans), drained
- salt and pepper

For the Topping
- 4 ounces wholewheat breadcrumbs
- $^1/_3$ cup Brazil nuts, chopped
- $^2/_3$ cup shredded half-fat cheddar cheese

Preheat the oven to 350°F.

Sauté the chopped leeks, garlic, and tomatoes in the oil until soft. Puree half the butter beans to a paste and add to the mixture. Season and add the remaining whole beans.

Transfer the mixture to an ovenproof dish and top with the combined breadcrumbs, nuts, and cheese. Cook in the oven for about 35–40 minutes.

Good source of **Allium** *vegetables, legumes, and selenium. Source of lycopene and vitamin E*
PER PORTION: 411 CAL, 18.5G FAT, 5.2G SATURATED FAT

butter bean casserole with cider

Serve this casserole with chunky wholewheat bread to mop up the delicious sauce. This dish has been selected from *The New Cranks Recipe Book* by Nadine Abensur.

SERVES 6

- 18 ounces fresh butter beans (or lima beans)
- 14 ounces onions, chopped
- 3 garlic cloves, crushed
- $^1/_3$ cup plus 1 tablespoon olive oil
- 9 ounces carrots, cut into 1-inch chunks
- dash of tamari (wheat-free soy sauce)
- $^1/_3$ cup plus 1 tablespoon hard cider
- 9 ounces zucchini, cut into 1-inch chunks
- 2½ cups button mushrooms
- 1¾ cups corn
- handful of fresh basil
- handful of fresh cilantro
- salt and freshly ground black pepper

Boil the fresh beans in plenty of water until they are tender but still intact. Drain and set aside, reserving some of the liquid. Meanwhile, in a large pot, heat the oil and sauté the onions and garlic until pale gold in color. Add the chunks of carrot and continue to sauté for a minute or 2, adding a little tamari and some of the cider. Then add the zucchini and sauté for another minute without letting them lose their color. Add the mushrooms, sauté for a few minutes, adding a little more tamari and a little more cider as well as salt and pepper, to taste. Finally add the corn and continue to stir.

Add the cooked butter beans with a little of the liquid they were cooked in and simmer gently for another 10 minutes, adding the remaining cider so that all the flavors come together.

Mix with plenty of fresh chopped basil and cilantro, and serve.

Good source of **Allium** *vegetables and legumes*
PER PORTION: 460 CAL, 18.8G FAT, 2.8G SATURATED FAT

sarah's pad thai

Pad Thai ("Thai-style frying") is a well-known Thai dish which is also very popular outside of Thailand. This version provides an alternative way to enjoy cruciferous and *Allium* vegetables by combining them with traditional Thai flavors. This recipe has been kindly provided by Sarah Dilley.

SERVES 4

- 2 tablespoons canola oil
- 3 eggs, beaten
- black pepper
- 9 ounces tofu, cut into ¾-inch cubes
- 4 garlic cloves, finely chopped
- 1 large red chile (optional)
- 14 ounces bok choy and/or other greens, chopped
- 3 scallions, cut into 1¼-inch strips
- 14 ounces pre-cooked rice noodles

- 7 ounces bean sprouts
- handful of peanuts
- lime wedges, for serving

For the Sauce
- 3 tablespoons oyster sauce
- 2 tablespoons fish sauce
- 2 tablespoons light soy sauce
- 1 tablespoon dark soy sauce (optional), plus extra for serving
- 1 tablespoon sugar

To make the sauce, simply combine all the sauce ingredients and set aside. Heat 1 tablespoon of the oil in a wok over high heat. Add the beaten eggs and pepper and swirl the pan so that the egg covers the bottom of it. Continue to swirl the pan and cook for about 3 minutes until the egg forms an omelet.

Slide a spatula around the side of the omelet to lift it from the sides of the pan, then flip it over—don't worry if it breaks. Transfer the omelet to a plate and chop into small pieces. Heat the second tablespoon of oil in the wok over medium–high heat. Stir-fry the tofu, garlic, and chile for 2 minutes. Add the bok choy or greens, and the scallions, and stir-fry for another 3 minutes.

Add the pre-cooked noodles and toss for 1 minute. Add the sauce and toss for a minute, then add the bean sprouts, chopped egg, and peanuts, and stir through. Serve with a lime wedge and dark soy sauce.

Good source of Allium *and cruciferous vegetables. Source of legumes, soy, and vitamin E*
PER PORTION: 418 CAL, 18.2G FAT, 2.3G SATURATED FAT

red lentil and caramelized onion and cabbage stuffed rolls

This lovely lunch dish was created by John Walter, Head Chef at the University of Surrey's Lakeside Restaurant. Serve the stuffed cabbage with a crunchy side salad, and Peanut and Flaxseed Bread (page 76).

SERVES 4

- ½ cup red lentils
- 8 large savoy cabbage leaves
- 1 large onion, cut in half and sliced
- 2 teaspoons olive oil
- 2 teaspoons demerara (or brown) sugar

- grated zest and juice of half a lemon
- freshly ground sea salt (or kosher salt) and black pepper

Preheat the oven to 350°F.

Wash the lentils, place in a saucepan, and cover with cold water. Cover the pan, bring to a boil, and skim off any foam. Boil rapidly for 10 minutes, stirring from time to time, then reduce to a simmer. Simmer for about 15 minutes, stirring and checking they are not burning or sticking to the bottom of the pan. The resulting consistency should be like oatmeal.

Wash and then blanch the cabbage leaves in boiling water for 2 minutes only, then refresh them in ice-cold water and let drain. Sauté the onion slices in olive oil over medium heat. When they start to brown, add the sugar and stir until nicely caramelized.

Combine the onions, cooked lentils, lemon juice and zest, and season to taste with salt and pepper. Put a heaping spoonful of the filling in the middle near the base of each leaf, fold over the sides of the cabbage leaf, and roll them up.

Put the stuffed cabbage rolls, seam sides down, in an oiled baking dish and brush lightly with olive oil. Bake for 20–25 minutes until lightly browned.

Source of Allium *vegetables, cruciferous vegetables, and legumes*
PER PORTION: 140 CAL, 2.6G FAT, 0.4G SATURATED FAT

pasta primavera

This pasta dish topped with a tasty vegetable sauce makes a filling lunch or evening meal. It has been adapted from a recipe in *Body and Beauty Foods* by Hazel Courteney and Kathryn Marsden.

SERVES 4

- 2 carrots, chopped
- 2 zucchinis, sliced
- 8 ounces small broccoli florets
- 4 ounces asparagus spears, cut into 1-inch lengths
- 6 ounces frozen peas
- 6–8 scallions, chopped
- 2 garlic cloves, crushed
- 16-oz. can diced tomatoes
- $^2/_3$ cup vegetable stock
- salt and pepper
- 1 tablespoon fresh parsley, chopped
- 1 tablespoon fresh basil, chopped
- 12 ounces wholewheat pasta spirals
- grated Parmesan cheese, for serving (optional)

Put the carrots, zucchini, broccoli, asparagus, peas, scallions, garlic, tomatoes, and stock in a large pot and bring to a boil, stirring occasionally. Reduce the heat, cover, and simmer for 10 minutes, stirring occasionally.

Uncover and cook for another 5–10 minutes until the vegetables are tender. Season to taste and stir in the herbs.

Meanwhile, cook the pasta according to the package instructions and drain. Spoon the pasta into pasta bowls and top with the sauce and a little Parmesan cheese, if you like.

Source of Allium *vegetables, cruciferous vegetables, legumes, lycopene, and vitamin E*
PER PORTION: 395 CAL, 4.2G FAT, 0.9G SATURATED FAT

potato pastry quiche

The potato pastry dough in this quiche is a surprisingly flavorsome, low-fat alternative to regular dough. The quiche can be made with roasted or fried vegetables. You could experiment with different vegetables, but ensure you pick some from the lists of beneficial foods. Serve with a leafy green salad. This recipe has been kindly provided by Kay Ford.

SERVES 4–6

For the Potato Pastry Dough
- 18 ounces potatoes (mixture of white and sweet), peeled and chopped
- 1¾ tablespoons olive oil spread
- ½ cup cornstarch

For the Filling
- 1 tablespoon olive oil
- 1 medium onion, red or white
- 3 garlic cloves, chopped
- 4 ounces broccoli, chopped into small florets
- ½ red chile, chopped
- ½ medium-size zucchini, sliced
- heaping ⅓ cup frozen peas
- ⅓ cup frozen corn
- 1½ cups sliced mushrooms
- 5 eggs, beaten
- 3½ tablespoons milk (soy milk)
- salt and pepper
- 1 tablespoon tomato paste
- 1 medium tomato, sliced
- a little blue cheese (optional)

Preheat the oven to 350°F.

Boil the potatoes for about 20 minutes or until soft. Drain and mash, with the olive oil spread and cornstarch. Grease a 12"-wide quiche pan and line with the potato mixture. Bake in the oven for 30–40 minutes. Set aside and let cool for at least an hour for the crust to set. (You could cook the pie shell a day ahead.)

Heat the oil in a frying pan over medium heat and cook all the vegetables except the tomato for 5 minutes. Meanwhile, beat the eggs together with the milk and salt and pepper.

Spread the tomato paste evenly over the pie shell, then fill with the vegetables and pour the egg mixture over them. Arrange the tomato slices on top and dot the blue cheese, if using, over that. Return to the oven for another 30 minutes.

Good source of Allium *vegetables. Source of cruciferous vegetables, lycopene, selenium, vitamin D, and vitamin E*
PER PORTION: 409 CAL, 18.7G FAT, 4.9G SATURATED FAT

cauliflower curry

This recipe was kindly provided by TV Chef Gino D'Acampo. Here's what he has to say about it:

"I have to admit that I'm not a big fan of curry, probably because it contains too many flavors and I'm not used to it, but whenever I have one, I tend to go for something mild and mainly vegetable based. Cauliflower works perfectly with the flavor of the curry paste, and the sweetness of the coconut milk balances the dish beautifully. I've tried this recipe with mixed vegetables and potatoes and it's fantastic."

SERVES 4

- 3 tablespoons olive oil
- 2 onions, finely chopped
- ½-inch piece ginger, peeled and grated
- 3 tablespoons curry paste
- 14-oz. can coconut milk
- 16-oz. can diced tomatoes
- 1 cauliflower, broken into pieces
- 2 potatoes, peeled and cut into ¾-inch chunks
- 3 tablespoons freshly squeezed lemon juice
- 7 ounces spinach leaves, washed
- salt, to taste

Heat the oil in a large pot and cook the onions for 5 minutes over medium heat until softened, stirring occasionally. Add the ginger and curry paste and continue to cook for 3 more minutes, stirring continuously.

Pour in the coconut milk and the chopped tomatoes and bring to a simmer. Add the cauliflower and the potatoes and cook for about 25 minutes or until the potatoes are softened. Season with salt and remove from the heat.

Add the lemon juice and spinach, cover, and leave for 2 minutes. Serve hot, just as it is, or to accompany one of your favorite main courses.

Good source of cruciferous vegetables. Source of **Allium** *vegetables, lycopene, and vitamin E*
PER PORTION: 301 CAL, 14.8G FAT, 2.0G SATURATED FAT

dr. john's omelet

This is best served with green vegetables or a green salad. You can also grate a small amount of cheese into the beaten eggs or add a handful of fresh chopped basil with the tomatoes. This recipe has been kindly provided by Dr. John Rayman.

SERVES 2

- 4 medium onions, or more to taste
- 1 tablespoon olive oil
- 12 cherry tomatoes, cut in half, or more to taste
- 5 eggs
- 2 tablespoons milk or soy milk
- handful of chopped chives (optional)

Preheat the broiler to hot.

Chop the onions and cook gently in olive oil in a large frying pan until soft and golden. Add the tomatoes and cook until just soft. Beat the eggs and milk in a bowl and add to the contents of the pan.

Cook gently, running a knife around the edge of the egg mixture to loosen it and to let the liquid run underneath. When the eggs are half cooked, put the frying pan under the hot broiler until the omelet has browned. Garnish with chives, if you like.

Good source of **Allium** *vegetables. Source of lycopene, selenium, vitamin D, and vitamin E*
PER PORTION: 414 CAL, 24.5G FAT, 6.0G SATURATED FAT

vegetarian chile

The use of Quorn (mycoprotein) makes for a delicious vegetarian alternative to beef in this classic Mexican-style dish. Serve with rice or crusty bread and "Chop-it-up" (Kushumb'r), page 147.

SERVES 6

- 1 tablespoon olive oil
- 1 medium–large onion, finely chopped
- 4 garlic cloves, finely chopped
- 1 tablespoon cumin
- 1 teaspoon ground coriander
- 1 red chile, finely chopped, or to taste
- 11 ounces frozen Quorn burger mix
- 2 x 16-oz. cans diced tomatoes
- 14½-oz. can Heinz baked beans
- 15-oz. can red kidney beans, drained
- salt and pepper
- ½ bunch of fresh cilantro, roughly chopped

Heat the oil in a large pot over medium heat, add the onion, and cook for 2–3 minutes. Add the garlic, spices, and chile, and cook gently for another 3 minutes.

Stir in the frozen Quorn mixture and 2–3 tablespoons of water and cook gently for about 5 minutes. Stir in the tomatoes, baked beans, kidney beans, and seasoning.

Cover, and simmer for 15 minutes, stirring occasionally. Finally, stir in the fresh cilantro and serve.

Good source of Allium *vegetables, legumes, and lycopene*
PER PORTION: 192 CAL, 5.2G FAT, 0.7G SATURATED FAT

stuffed peppers

The peanuts give this dish a lovely nutty flavor. Grains such as bulgur or rice can be used instead for the stuffing. A sprinkle of strong cheese in the last ten minutes of cooking adds a tasty topping. This dish has been kindly provided by Tracy Forward.

SERVES 2

- ½ cup couscous
- 1 cup boiling water
- 2 large peppers
- 1 tablespoon olive oil, plus a little extra for drizzling
- 1 large onion, chopped
- 1 garlic clove, chopped
- 1 ounce sun-dried tomatoes in oil, drained and chopped
- 3 tablespoons unsalted peanuts
- 1 tablespoon sunflower seeds
- 2 large handfuls of arugula
- 1–2 tablespoons sweet chile sauce

Preheat the oven to 350°F.

Put the couscous in a saucepan and pour the boiling water over it. Return to a boil and cook for a minute while stirring. Turn off the heat and let the couscous swell for about 5 minutes.

Cut the peppers in half through the stalks, remove the seeds, and place them in an ovenproof dish. Gently heat the oil in a frying pan and cook the onion and garlic for about 5 minutes until golden brown. Add the tomatoes, peanuts, and sunflower seeds, and continue cooking for 1 minute.

Stir in the arugula and cook for a minute or so until it has wilted. Stir in the prepared couscous and chile sauce to taste. Pile the mixture into the pepper halves, press down, and drizzle with a little extra olive oil. Cover and cook for about 45 minutes or until the peppers are tender. Remove the cover for the last 10 minutes of cooking.

Good source of Allium *vegetables. Source of cruciferous vegetables, lycopene, and vitamin E*
PER PORTION: 526 CAL, 34.9G FAT, 4.9G SATURATED FAT

simple tomato sauce

This versatile sauce can be used with pasta, meat, poultry, fish, or vegetables. It can be made with dried mixed herbs instead of fresh basil—just add two teaspoons dried herbs when cooking the onion and garlic. The sauce can be blended to a smooth consistency if you prefer.

SERVES 4

- 1 tablespoon olive oil
- 1 large onion, finely chopped
- 4 garlic cloves, crushed
- 2 x 16-oz. cans diced tomatoes
- ¼ cup tomato paste
- 2 teaspoons sugar
- handful of fresh basil, chopped

Heat the oil in a pot and gently cook the onion and garlic until soft.

Add the tomatoes, tomato paste, and sugar, and simmer for about 20 minutes, adding a little water if the mixture becomes too thick.

Add the fresh basil and cook for another couple of minutes.

Good source of Allium *vegetables and lycopene. Source of vitamin E*
PER PORTION: 123 CAL, 4.0G FAT, 1.0G SATURATED FAT

broccoli and fava bean frittata

Frittatas are a great way of using up leftover vegetables to make a filling meal in minutes. Do include vegetables that are particularly beneficial.

SERVES 2

- 1½ tablespoons olive oil spread
- 1 medium onion, sliced
- 4 ounces potato, boiled and sliced or chopped
- 1½ cups broccoli florets, cooked
- ¾ cup kale, cooked
- ¾ cup fava beans, cooked
- 4 eggs
- salt and pepper

Preheat the broiler to hot.

Melt the spread in a frying pan. Add the onion and sauté until soft. Add the potato and continue cooking until golden brown.

Add the remaining vegetables and heat through. Meanwhile, whisk together the eggs and season with salt and pepper. Add the egg mixture to the vegetables and stir gently.

Let the frittata set for a minute or so, then place the frying pan under a hot broiler to brown the top.

Source of **Allium** *and cruciferous vegetables, legumes, selenium, vitamin D, and vitamin E*
PER PORTION: 329 CAL, 19.9G FAT, 5.4G SATURATED FAT

vegetable sides

braised red cabbage

This colorful dish makes a wonderful sweet-and-sour accompaniment to poultry, pork, or game. The flavor benefits from the long, slow cooking time. This dish has been adapted from a recipe by Jane Baxter.

SERVES 6

- 1¼ pounds red cabbage, shredded
- 9 ounces onions, finely chopped
- 2 cooking apples, peeled, cored, and finely chopped
- 2 garlic cloves, finely chopped
- ½ cup currants
- 1 teaspoon ground allspice
- 1 tablespoon brown sugar
- 1 tablespoon red wine vinegar
- 1 tablespoon olive oil spread
- salt and pepper

Preheat the oven to 300°F.

Arrange a layer of cabbage in the bottom of a large casserole dish. Add a layer of onions, apples, garlic, currants, spices, sugar, and salt and pepper. Continue to alternate the layers until all the ingredients are used.

Pour the wine vinegar over them and dot with the olive oil spread. Cover the dish with foil and bake slowly in the oven for 1½–2 hours.

Good source of cruciferous vegetables. Source of **Allium** *vegetables*
PER PORTION: 71 CAL, 2G FAT, 0.4G SATURATED FAT

baked shallots

This side dish makes a great accompaniment to a roast dinner; it has been adapted from a recipe by Jane Baxter.

SERVES 6

- 18 ounces shallots, peeled
- 1 tablespoon olive oil spread
- salt and pepper
- 1 tablespoon sugar
- ½ cup red wine

Preheat the oven to 300°F.

Arrange the peeled shallots in a single layer in a shallow flameproof and ovenproof pan. Dot with the olive oil spread and season to taste with salt and pepper. Cook over a medium heat until browned.

Sprinkle with sugar and cook until the sugar disappears. Add the red wine and bring to a boil and cover. Bake in the oven for about 15 minutes until tender.

Good source of **Allium** *vegetables*
PER PORTION: 52 CAL, 1.5G FAT, 0.3G SATURATED FAT

moonblush tomatoes

This is one of Nigella Lawson's recipes. She invented it as a delicious alternative to buying sunblush (semi-dried) tomatoes. The name refers to the way they are left to cook throughout the night. They can be served in any number of ways —with bread or cheese, as part of a salad or as a pasta sauce.

SERVES 5

- 18 ounces (about 24) on-the-vine cherry or other baby tomatoes
- 2 teaspoons kosher salt (or 1 tablespoon table salt)
- ¼ teaspoon sugar
- 1 teaspoon dried thyme
- 2 tablespoons olive oil

Preheat the oven to 425°F.

Cut the tomatoes in half and sit them, cut side up, in an ovenproof dish. Sprinkle with the salt, sugar, thyme, and olive oil. Place in the hot oven and immediately turn it off. Leave the tomatoes in the oven overnight or for a whole day, without opening the door.

Source of lycopene
PER PORTION: 66.8 CAL, 5.6G FAT, 0.8G SATURATED FAT

roasted tomatoes on the vine

Serving the tomatoes still on the vine makes an attractive and delicious side dish.

SERVES 2

- 7 ounces cherry or other tomatoes, on the vine
- 1 teaspoon olive oil
- salt and pepper

Preheat the oven to 400°F.

Brush the tomatoes, still on the vine, with the olive oil and sprinkle with salt and pepper. Roast in the oven for 20–25 minutes.

Source of lycopene
PER PORTION: 32 CAL, 1.9G FAT, 0.3G SATURATED FAT

chop-it-up (kushumb'r)

Chop-it-up is named as such simply because that's all you need to do with each ingredient. It makes a refreshing chutney to accompany spicy dishes. This recipe has been kindly provided by Mrs. John Dilley.

SERVES 4

- ½ English cucumber
- 2 tomatoes
- 1 medium onion
- 1 tablespoon lime juice
- lettuce, shredded (optional)
- chile, finely chopped (optional)

Cut the cucumber, tomatoes, and onion by hand into cubes of uniform size and mix together. Stir in the lime juice and the lettuce, and chile, if using. You may remove the seeds and peel from the cucumber, if you like.

Source of Allium *vegetables and lycopene*
PER PORTION: 29 CAL, 0.3G FAT, 0.1G SATURATED FAT

gujarati cabbage

This dish makes an ideal accompaniment to curries. Any type of cabbage will do, but Savoy is best. This dish has been adapted from a recipe by Jane Baxter.

SERVES 4

- 1 tablespoon vegetable oil
- 1 tablespoon black mustard seeds
- 1 dried chile
- ½ cabbage, thinly sliced
- 2 carrots, coarsely grated
- 1 tablespoon sugar
- juice of half a lemon
- salt and pepper, to taste

Heat the oil in a large wok until hot and add the mustard seeds and chile. When the seeds start to pop, add the cabbage and carrots and stir-fry for 5 minutes.

Add the remaining ingredients and season to taste. Cook for another minute and serve immediately.

Good source of cruciferous vegetables
PER PORTION: 108 CAL, 4.3G FAT, 0.5G SATURATED FAT

dal

This delicious dal is lovely with nan bread or rice. Alternatively, it can be served as an accompaniment to your favorite curry.

SERVES 4

- 2 tablespoons olive oil
- 1 medium onion, chopped
- 3 garlic cloves, crushed
- 1 red chile pepper, sliced
- 1 teaspoon ground turmeric
- 3 teaspoons garam masala
- 1 teaspoon cumin seeds
- ½-inch piece fresh ginger, peeled
- 1⅔ cups split red lentils, rinsed
- 2 medium tomatoes, chopped
- 2 tablespoons fresh cilantro, chopped
- salt and pepper

Heat the oil in a large pot and gently cook the onion, garlic, and chile pepper until they just start to brown. Add the turmeric, garam masala, cumin seeds, and ginger, and cook for another 2 minutes.

Add the lentils and pour in 4 cups of boiling water. Bring the lentils to a boil and simmer for 15–20 minutes or until they are soft.

Add the tomatoes and cook for another 5 minutes. Stir in the cilantro, season to taste with salt and pepper, and serve.

Good source of **Allium** *vegetables and legumes. Source of lycopene*
PER PORTION: 337 CAL, 8.8G FAT, 1.2G SATURATED FAT

chickpea mash

Chickpea mash is a great alternative to mashed potatoes, and it can be ready in five minutes.

SERVES 2

- 15-oz. can chickpeas, drained
- black pepper
- 2 teaspoons olive oil
- 1 tablespoon chopped fresh parsley

Gently heat the drained chickpeas in a pan of water over a low heat for a few minutes and drain. There is no need to boil them as they are already cooked.

Grind in the pepper, to taste, and mash the chickpeas with a potato masher. Finally, stir in the olive oil and parsley.

Good source of legumes
PER PORTION: 180 CAL, 8.0G FAT, 1.0G SATURATED FAT

moros y cristianos (black beans with white rice)

This recipe is another reminder of the Moors' place in Spanish history, a visual as well as a culinary reference with the black beans and white rice. Moros y Cristianos can be served with roast duck. This recipe was taken from *Moro: The Cookbook* by Sam and Sam Clark.

SERVES 4

- 1 cup black beans, soaked overnight
- ½ medium onion
- 2 garlic cloves
- 2 bay leaves, preferably fresh
- ½ cinnamon stick
- juice and zest of half an orange
- 3 tablespoons olive oil
- ½ small bunch of fresh flat-leaf parsley, roughly chopped
- ¾ cup short-grain white rice (Calasparra)
- sea salt (or kosher salt) and black pepper

Drain the beans and place in a large pot with at least 6 cups of cold water. Add the onion, garlic, bay leaves, and cinnamon stick.

Cook for 1–2 hours, until soft, scooping off any foam that forms on top. Season with salt and pepper, add the orange zest, orange juice, olive oil, and parsley, and set aside.

Simmer the rice in lightly salted boiling water until firm but not chalky (about 10–15 minutes), and drain. When you are ready, serve the rice, then spoon the beans and a little of their juices on top so you can see both the black and white.

Good source of legumes. Source of Allium *vegetables*
PER PORTION: 359 CAL, 10.6G FAT, 1.5G SATURATED FAT

broccoli saltati

This Italian-style broccoli stir-fry was kindly provided by Gino D'Acampo. Here is what he has to say about it:

"Everybody in my family loves broccoli and we always have it in the house. One day I thought I would experiment with a few Oriental ingredients. This is what came out of that day."

SERVES 6

- 1 tablespoon plus ¼ cup olive oil
- 2 tablespoons honey
- 1 tablespoon light soy sauce
- 2 tablespoons balsamic vinegar
- 1 garlic clove, finely sliced
- 1 small red chile, seeded and finely sliced
- 3 tablespoons sliced fresh basil leaves
- ½ cup pine nuts
- 1½ pounds broccoli, cut into florets
- salt and pepper

In a large bowl, mix together 1 tablespoon of the olive oil, the honey, soy sauce, balsamic vinegar, garlic, chile, basil, and pine nuts in a large bowl.

Bring a large pot of salted water to a boil and cook the broccoli for 3 minutes until *al dente*. Drain the broccoli and place in the bowl with the dressing. Toss gently to avoid breaking up the broccoli.

Heat the remaining olive oil in a wok and fry the broccoli with its dressing for 4 minutes until piping hot, stirring frequently. Adjust the seasoning and serve as an accompaniment to fish or meat.

Good source of cruciferous vegetables. Source of vitamin E
PER PORTION: 240 CAL, 19.6G FAT, 2.4G SATURATED FAT

sweet potato boulangère

Sweet potatoes make a great change to ordinary potatoes in this classic dish.

SERVES 6

- 2 pounds sweet potatoes, peeled and sliced
- 1 large onion, peeled and sliced
- 3 garlic cloves, crushed
- 2½ cups hot chicken stock
- 1 teaspoon dried mixed herbs
- 1 teaspoon dried thyme

Preheat the oven to 400°F.

Put the potatoes, onion, and garlic into a large pot and pour in the hot stock. Add the herbs and bring to a boil for 10 minutes.

Pour into an ovenproof dish and place in the oven for about 45 minutes or until there is only a small amount of liquid left.

Good source of Allium *vegetables. Source of vitamin E*
PER PORTION: 152 CAL, 0.9G FAT, 0.2G SATURATED FAT

desserts

berry and nut crumble

This is a delicious crumble with a wonderfully different topping. To make it a source or good source of the particularly beneficial polyphenols, simply substitute raspberries for some or all of the mixed berries.

SERVES 6

- 18 ounces frozen mixed berries, defrosted
- 3 tablespoons sugar

For the Crumble Topping
- heaping ¾ cup flour
- ½ cup soy spread
- 1 cup rolled oats
- ½ cup Brazil nuts, chopped
- scant ½ cup sugar
- pinch of salt

Preheat the oven to 400°F.

Put the fruit in an ovenproof dish and sprinkle with the sugar.

Put the flour and soy spread in a bowl and rub in the spread until it resembles fine breadcrumbs. Add the remaining ingredients and mix well.

Spread the crumble mixture over the fruit and bake for about 30 minutes or until the top is golden.

Good source of selenium. Source of vitamin D and vitamin E
PER PORTION: 418 CAL, 19.6G FAT, 4.7G SATURATED FAT

winter fruit salad

This is a wonderful, warm dessert which tastes excellent with a little soy ice cream. You could try varying the dried fruit. This recipe has been kindly provided by Sylvia Wainwright.

SERVES 6

- 2 cups pitted prunes
- 1⅔ cups dried apricots
- 1⅔ cups dried peaches
- 2 cooking apples, peeled and sliced
- 2 green tea bags

Place all the ingredients in a pan. Add barely enough water to cover the fruit and simmer for about 10 minutes.

Let cool and remove the tea bags.

Source of polyphenols
PER PORTION: 254 CAL, 0.9G FAT, 0.0G SATURATED FAT

pomegranate upside-down cake

This is a new take on an old classic and is perfect for a cold autumn afternoon with a warm cup of green tea.

SERVES 8

For the Topping
- 2 cups pomegranate juice
- 11 ounces pomegranate arils
- 2 tablespoons sugar

For the Sponge Cake
- ¾ cup olive oil spread
- ¾ cup sugar
- 3 eggs
- 1⅓ cups flour, sifted
- 1½ teaspoons baking powder
- ⅛ teaspoon salt
- 3 tablespoons milk
- 2 tablespoons of orange or lemon juice or a teaspoon of vanilla extract

Preheat the oven to 350°F.

Gently reduce the pomegranate juice in a nonstick pan with a heavy bottom over a low–medium heat until it turns into syrup. Stir occasionally and do not let it boil as this will cause the sugars to caramelize and set hard. As the juice reduces, adjust the heat accordingly, until there are only about 4 or 5 tablespoons left; this will take up to about 50 minutes.

Meanwhile, make the cake batter. Cream the olive oil spread and sugar together in a large mixing bowl. Whisk in the eggs with a couple of tablespoons of the flour. Then fold in the remaining flour and dry ingredients. Finally mix, in the milk and fruit juice or vanilla extract.

Line an 8-inch cake pan with parchment paper or grease the pan. Ladle in the pomegranate syrup and spread evenly over the bottom. Sprinkle the sugar over it, then cover with all but a handful of the arils in an even layer. Spoon the cake batter over the fruit and smooth the top. Bake in the oven for 45–50 minutes or until a skewer stuck into the middle comes out clean). Let the cake cool for 5 minutes.

Tip the cake out onto a rack and cool for 20 minutes. Upside-down cake is best served when still warm. Sprinkle the reserved pomegranate arils around the plate to decorate.

Good source of polyphenols
PER PORTION: 378 CAL, 16.6G FAT, 3.3G SATURATED FAT

summer fruits in red wine, monbazillac, basil, and mint

This wonderfully subtle recipe was kindly provided by chef Raymond Blanc's kitchen. It is perfect for a summer's day with the refreshing taste of red fruits combined with a hint of mint and basil. Other fruits can be used (blackberries, blueberries, or peaches). If the fruit is not ripe enough, you can marinate it in a little sugar for an hour. This dessert can be prepared 4–6 hours in advance.

SERVES 4

- 1 cup Monbazillac or other dessert wine
- ½ cup red wine (cabernet sauvignon)
- 3 tablespoons sugar
- ½ vanilla bean, seeds scraped out and set aside
- 12 leaves fresh mint, lightly chopped
- 6 leaves fresh basil, lightly chopped
- 2 cups raspberries
- 1½ cups strawberries, stemmed and quartered
- ⅓ cup wild strawberries (optional)
- 1 large wedge of watermelon, peeled, seeded, and cubed or made into balls
- ½ cup chilled pink champagne (optional, but the remainder will be very much appreciated by your guests)

Bring the two wines, sugar, vanilla bean and seeds to a boil in a pan. Boil to remove the alcohol and then turn off the heat. Tie the herbs up in a muslin bag and add to the pan to infuse the liquid. Cool down to about 105°F so that the fruit does not cook and lose its shape when it's added.

Add the raspberries, strawberries, and the melon, and refrigerate for at least 4 hours.

Remove the herbs and vanilla bean, and place the cold fruit soup into a large serving bowl or 4 individual bowls. Pour about 2 tablespoons of the pink champagne, if using, over the top as you are serving.

Good source of lycopene. Source of polyphenols
PER PORTION: 193 CAL, 0.5G FAT, 0.2G SATURATED FAT

watermelon sherbet

This sherbet is a beautiful pink color and has a refreshing taste.

SERVES 4

- ⅓ cup pomegranate juice (or water)
- 6 tablespoons sugar
- ½ watermelon
- juice of half a lemon

Heat the pomegranate juice or water, and the sugar in a pan over medium heat, stirring occasionally. Heat for a few minutes until the sugar has dissolved; there is no need to boil. Remove from the heat and chill in the fridge.

Remove and discard the seeds from the watermelon. Scoop out the flesh and blend in a blender with the lemon juice until smooth. Mix the watermelon puree with the pomegranate and sugar mixture. Churn and freeze the sherbet mixture in an ice cream maker following the manufacturer's instructions.

Alternatively, pour into a freezer-proof container and place in the freezer. Leave it for an hour, allowing the mixture to start freezing. Remove from the freezer and beat with beaters to break up the ice, then replace in the freezer. Repeat this several times until the sherbet is frozen. This will take up to about 5 hours.

Good source of lycopene
PER PORTION: 122 CAL, 0.4G FAT, 0.1G SATURATED FAT

crêpes with raspberry sauce

These crêpes make an attractive dessert and are also ideal for a special breakfast.

SERVES 4

- ⅔ cup plain flour
- 1 egg, lightly beaten
- 1 cup soy milk
- 1½ tablespoons olive oil spread, melted
- pinch of salt
- extra fat spread for greasing the pan

For the Sauce
- 18 ounces raspberries
- 1 teaspoon brown sugar
- confectioners' sugar for dusting

Place the flour in a large bowl and whisk in the egg, milk, fat spread, and salt until the batter is smooth. Chill in the fridge for 1 hour.

Preheat the oven to 250°F.

While the batter is chilling, set aside a few raspberries for each portion. Place half the remaining raspberries into a saucepan with a teaspoon of water and sprinkle the brown sugar over them. Cook the raspberries over medium heat for about 5 minutes, breaking them up with a wooden spoon. Reduce the heat and let the sauce thicken; this will take about 5 minutes.

Add the other half of the raspberries and gently heat until they are warmed through but whole. Grease a nonstick frying pan with a little spread and place over medium heat. Ladle about 3 tablespoons of the batter into the pan and swirl it so that it is covered with a thin layer of batter. Cook for about a minute, running a spatula around the edge of the crêpe to lift it away from the edges. Shake the pan to loosen the crêpe and flip it over. When cooked, transfer to a plate and keep warm in the oven while you cook the rest of the crêpes.

Lay a crêpe on a plate and spoon some of the sauce onto it. Fold a third from one side into the middle, then a third from the other side. Repeat until you've done this to 8 crêpes. Dust with confectioners' sugar and garnish with a few of the reserved raspberries.

Good source of polyphenols. Source of soy
PER PORTION: 215 CAL, 9.0G FAT, 2.8G SATURATED FAT

dairy-free chocolate ice cream

This delicious dessert was devised by John Walter, Head Chef at the University of Surrey's Lakeside Restaurant. He originally created it for his son who has a milk allergy. If you have a sweet tooth, go for a sweeter dark chocolate as some dark chocolate can be quite bitter.

SERVES 6

- 11 ounces dairy-free dark chocolate, broken into squares, plus extra for garnishing
- 2 cups soy cream for garnishing

Place both the chocolate and soy cream in a microwaveable bowl. Microwave on the defrost setting for 3 minutes or until the chocolate has melted. Stir well.

Pour the mixture into a freezer-proof container and freeze for about 2 hours. Remove the ice cream from the freezer and beat until smooth.

Return to the freezer for a couple of hours or until the ice cream has set. (If you have an ice cream maker, you can use this instead.) Scoop into bowls and add a piece of dark chocolate when ready to serve.

Source of soy
PER PORTION: 367 CAL, 26.8G FAT, 12.4G SATURATED FAT

chocolate-raspberry cups

These chocolate cups are smooth and creamy and blend beautifully with the fresh raspberries. The recipe has been selected from www.alprosoya.co.uk.

SERVES 4

- 3½-oz. bar luxury Belgian dark chocolate
- 12 white marshmallows, chopped
- 1 cup fresh raspberries
- 1 cup chocolate-flavored soy milk

Break the chocolate into squares, place with the marshmallows in the top of a double boiler set over simmering water, and let them melt. Place enough raspberries in each ramekin dish to cover the bottoms.

Whisk together the chocolate-flavored soy milk with the melted chocolate mixture and pour into the individual ramekins, over the raspberries.

Chill for 2 hours and serve decorated with a couple of fresh raspberries and a sprig of mint.

Source of polyphenols and soy
PER PORTION: 231 CAL, 8.5G FAT, 4.5G SATURATED FAT

ruby fruit salad with raspberry coulis

This is a pretty and refreshing dessert that is very simple to make.

SERVES 4

- 4 ounces pomegranate arils
- 4 ounces watermelon, cubed
- 4 ounces red seedless grapes
- 1 cup raspberries

For the Coulis
- 1¼ cups raspberries
- juice of half a lime
- 3 tablespoons confectioners' sugar

Combine the fruit and place in 1 large or 4 individual serving dishes.

Mix the raspberries with the lime juice and sugar and blend to make a smooth puree. Drizzle the coulis over the fruit and serve.

Good source of polyphenols. Source of lycopene
PER PORTION: 259 CAL, 1.3G FAT, 0.3G SATURATED FAT

pomegranate sherbet

The sharp, tangy flavors of the pomegranate and lime combine in this vibrant sherbet to make an irresistible dessert.

SERVES 4

- ⅓ cup water
- ⅓ cup sugar
- 2 cups pomegranate juice
- juice of half a lime

Heat the water and sugar in a pan over medium heat for a few minutes, stirring occasionally until the sugar has dissolved (there is no need to boil). Remove from the heat and chill in the fridge.

Mix the pomegranate and lime juices with the water and sugar mixture. Churn and freeze the sherbet mixture in an ice cream maker following the manufacturer's instructions.

Alternatively, pour into a freezer-proof container and place in the freezer. Leave it for an hour, allowing the mixture to start freezing. Remove from the freezer and beat with a beater to break up the ice, then replace in the freezer.

Repeat this several times until the sherbet is frozen. This will take up to 7 hours.

Good source of polyphenols
PER PORTION: 127 CAL, 0.0G FAT, 0.0G SATURATED FAT

raspberry and brazil nut muffins

These muffins have a lovely nutty bite and can be quite addictive. They freeze well and can be gently warmed in the microwave.

MAKES 12 MUFFINS

- 2 medium eggs
- ¾ cup sugar
- ¼ cup canola oil
- ¾ cup soy milk
- 1⅓ cups white flour, sifted
- ⅔ cup wholewheat flour, sifted
- 1 cup rolled oats
- 1 tablespoon baking powder
- 2 x 10-ounce cans raspberries in fruit juice, drained
- ½ cup Brazil nuts, roughly chopped

Preheat the oven to 375°F.

Place 12 paper muffin cups in a 12-cup muffin pan. Beat together the eggs and sugar until pale and fluffy. Add the oil and milk and continue to beat until incorporated. Add all the dry ingredients and fold in.

Finally, add the raspberries and Brazil nuts and fold in. Pour the mixture into the paper muffin cups and bake for 25–30 minutes until well risen and golden brown.

Good source of selenium. Source of polyphenols
PER MUFFIN: 262 CAL, 10.4G FAT, 1.5G SATURATED FAT

glossary

5-alpha-dihydroxytestosterone: A more potent product of the male sex hormone testosterone.

Androgen receptor: By binding to the androgen receptor, the androgen hormones, testosterone, and dihydrotestosterone turn on genes to produce proteins that are responsible for male characteristics and control the behavior of cells.

Androgen-insensitive cells: Cells that no longer react to androgens.

Androgens: A group of male sex hormones including testosterone and dihydrotestosterone.

Anti-atherogenic: Helps prevent atherosclerosis (see later entry).

Antimicrobial: A substance that either prevents the growth of or kills bacteria.

Antioxidant: A substance, such as vitamin E, vitamin C, or beta carotene, thought to protect body cells from the damaging effects of oxidation (see later entry).

Atherosclerosis: The build-up of fatty deposits in the arteries.

Blood vessels: Tubular vessels including arteries and veins that transport blood around the body.

Cancer cells: Cells that have become cancerous.

Cell division: A process whereby a cell divides into new cells.

Detoxification: The process of making a harmful substance less toxic.

Diallyl disulphide (DADS): An organosulphur compound produced by *Allium* vegetables.

DNA: Deoxyribonucleic acid—a double helix structure that contains the genetic information required to direct the development and functioning of all living organisms.

Enzyme: A protein that speeds up the rate of a chemical reaction.

Estrogen receptor-beta: A receptor located on DNA that is activated by estrogen that can turn on genes regulating the production of proteins and resulting in a change in cell function.

Fatty acid: A basic component of fats and oils released during digestion. The type of fatty acid determines the properties of dietary fat (e.g., solid or oil) and the structure of cell membranes.

Gene: A section of DNA (genetic material) that provides the instructions for the creation of a specific protein.

Gleason score: A score (between two and ten) based upon the appearance of prostate tissue (how well organized it is) under the microscope; cancers with a higher Gleason score are more aggressive.

Goitrogen: A substance that inhibits the uptake of iodine from the diet and interferes with thyroid function.

Hormone: A substance that is made in one part of the body and is released into the bloodstream so that it can travel to the organs or body tissues and interact with an appropriate receptor; a hormone triggers a change in the structure or function of its target.

Hormone-dependent disease: Prostate cancer which requires androgens, particularly the hormone testosterone, in order to grow.

Hormone-independent disease: Prostate cancer which has adapted so that it no longer needs androgens in order to grow.

Immune function: A number of processes that help to protect the body from disease.

Immune response: The response of the body to a harmful invader, e.g., an infective agent or cancer cells.

Inflammation: A localised protective reaction of tissue to irritation, injury, or infection, characterized by pain, redness, swelling, and sometimes loss of function.

Insulin-like growth-factor-1: A hormone that stimulates growth.

Locally advanced disease: Prostate cancer that has spread beyond the prostate gland into the surrounding tissue.

Metabolite: A product or intermediate product of a set of chemical reactions in the body.

Metastatic: When a cancer spreads from its original site to another area of the body it is called metastasis.

Nutrients: Substances that are typically eaten and provide the materials for growth and energy or help regulate these processes. Examples of macronutrients are carbohydrate, protein, and fat, and examples of micronutrients are vitamins and minerals, such as vitamin C and selenium.

Estrogen (Oestrogen): A female sex hormone that promotes the formation of female characteristics.

Oxidation: An interaction with oxygen. PUFAs (polyunsaturated fatty acids) may undergo oxidation inside the body which, when excessive, may result in harmful effects.

Oxidative stress: A condition of increased oxidant production in animal cells characterized by the release of harmful substances that result in damage to cells.

Pre-cancerous: A condition that, if left untreated, may result in cancer.

PSA: Prostate Specific Antigen —a protein that is produced by the prostate gland and is often elevated in prostate cancer. Elevated PSA levels can be detected with a blood test and provide an indicator for prostate cancer diagnosis and progression.

PSA doubling time: The period of time that it takes for a PSA level to double. The shorter the doubling time, the more aggressive the cancer is likely to be, so it is used as an indicator of prostate cancer progression.

Stage III or IV prostate cancer: At stage III, cancer has spread beyond the outer layer of the prostate to nearby tissues. At stage IV, cancer has spread to other parts of the body, such as the bladder, rectum, bone, liver, lungs, and lymph nodes.

Status: A description of deficiency, adequacy, or excess of a nutrient.

Testosterone: A male sex hormone that promotes the formation of male characteristics.

Tumor: A swelling that is formed by the abnormal growth of cells such as cancer cells.

The following recipes and variations of recipes have been reprinted by kind permission:

Oatmeal with raspberry and pomegranate compote: adapted from a recipe on www.alprosoya.co.uk

Bagels with oven-roasted tomatoes and arugula: taken from www.eggrecipes.co.uk

Watercress soup: adapted from a recipe on www.alprosoya.co.uk

POM salsa: recipe selected from www.pomwonderful.com

Tuna stir-fry: adapted from a recipe on www.sainsburys.co.uk/food

POM vinaigrette: recipe from www.pomwonderful.com

POM stuffed halibut: adapted from a recipe on www.pomwonderful.com

Turkey and apricot casserole: adapted from a recipe on www.sainsburys.co.uk/food

Spicy bean pita: adapted from a recipe in Morrison's *Let's Eat Smart* magazine (January/February 2008)

Baked shallots, Braised red cabbage, Gujarati cabbage: adapted from recipes by Jane Baxter on www.riverford.co.uk

Chocolate-raspberry cups: recipe selected from www.alprosoya.co.uk

The recipes and variations of recipes below have been selected from the following cookbooks and reprinted by kind permission of the publishers:

From *Arabesque* by Claudia Roden, Penguin Books Limited, reprinted by kind permission of David Higham Associates:

Shrimp in spicy tomato sauce
Stuffed eggplant

From *Body and Beauty Foods* by Hazel Courteney and Kathryn Marsden, published by Ivy Press:
Pasta Primavera
Sweet and sour turkey meatballs
Fettuccine with salmon, zucchini, and almonds

From *Cooking with the Kosher Butcher's Wife* by Sharon Lurie, published by Struik (2006):
Liver and onions

From *Gordon Ramsay Makes it Easy* by Gordon Ramsay, published by Quadrille (2005):
Tiger shrimp salad with mango and avocado

From *Moro: the Cookbook* by Sam and Sam Clark, published by Ebury. Reprinted by permission of The Random House Group Ltd:
Fava bean puree
Moros y cristianos

From *Nigella Express* by Nigella Lawson, published by Chatto & Windus. Reprinted by permission of The Random House Group Ltd:
Moonblush tomatoes

From *The New Cranks Recipe Book* by Nadine Abensur, published by Weidenfeld & Nicolson, reprinted by kind permission from Cranks:
Butter bean casserole
Caribbean pepperpot
Cauliflower and broccoli salad

The following recipes were kindly provided by celebrity chefs. For further information see their websites, listed below:

Alex Mackay, www.alexmackay.com
Tiger shrimp and shiitake mushroom broth
Sea-bream (porgy) with sunblush tomatoes and basil

Antony Worrall Thompson, www.awtonline.co.uk
Chilled tomato bisque
Spicy sardines with chickpea and avocado salad

Cyrus Todiwala, www.cafespice.co.uk
Saag aloo with oily fish
Stuffed duck breast (Badak chaanti badami pasanda)
Jardaloo ma murghi

Gino D'Acampo, www.ginodacampo.com
Cauliflower curry
Broccoli saltati

Raymond Blanc, www.raymondblanc.com
Summer fruits in red wine, Monbazillac, basil, and mint
Poached salmon steak on spinach and watercress puree

Details of the University of Surrey's Lakeside Restaurant can be found on:
www.som.surrey.ac.uk/about/lakeside/index.asp
Head chef John Walter kindly provided the following recipes:

Deviled mackerel with tomato and mint salad
Trout and leek paupiette in carrot and coriander sauce
Red lentil and caramelized-onion stuffed cabbage rolls
Dairy-free ice cream

The following recipes were provided by Dr. John Rayman (additional recipes credited throughout the book):

Dr. John's meatballs
Stir-fried pork tenderloin
Peanut and flaxseed bread

index

resources

Prostate Cancer Foundation
1250 Fourth Street
Santa Monica, CA 90401
1-800-757-CURE (2873)
www.prostatecancer.org

American Cancer Society
Man-to-Man Program
1-800-227-2345
www.cancer.org

Cancer Care
275 Seventh Avenue
New York, NY 10001
1-800-813-4673
www.cancercare.org

National Cancer Institute
6116 Executive Boulevard
Bethesda, MD 20892
1-800-422-6237
www.cancer.gov

U.S. Department of Health & Human Services
200 Independence Avenue, S.W.
Washington, D.C. 20201
1-877-696-6775
www.healthfinder.gov

USDA Food and Nutrition Information Center
National Agricultural Library
10301 Baltimore Avenue, Room 105
Beltsville, MD 20705
301-504-5414
www.nutrition.gov

Centers for Disease Control and Prevention
1600 Clifton Road
Atlanta, GA 30333
1-800-CDC-INFO (1-800-232-4636)
www.cdc.gov

Canadian Prostate Cancer Network
P.O. Box 1253
Lakefield, ON
K0L 2H0
Canada
1-866-810-2726
www.cpcn.org

Prostate Cancer Research Foundation of Canada
145 Front Street, Suite 306
Toronto, ON
M5A 1E3
Canada
1-888-255-0333
www.prostatecancer.ca

Would you like to help with our research?
Researchers at the Food, Consumer Behaviour, and
Health Research Centre at the University of Surrey are
interested in your views on food, prostate health, and how
you view this cookbook. Please log onto our website
(www.fahs.surrey.ac.uk/survey/prostatecarecookbook/)
and complete a short questionnaire.